Suggestible

YOU

Suggestible Y⊙U

Placebos, False Memories, Hypnosis, *and the* Power *of* Your Astonishing Brain

Erik Vance

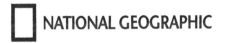

NATIONAL GEOGRAPHIC

Washington, D.C.

Published by National Geographic Partners, LLC
1145 17th Street NW, Washington, DC 20036

Library of Congress Cataloging-in-Publication Data
ISBN: 978-1-4262-1789-0

Since 1888, the National Geographic Society has funded more than 12,000 research, exploration, and preservation projects around the world. National Geographic Partners distributes a portion of the funds it receives from your purchase to National Geographic Society to support programs including the conservation of animals and their habitats.

National Geographic Partners
1145 17th Street NW
Washington, DC 20036-4688 USA

Become a member of National Geographic and activate your benefits today at natgeo .com/jointoday.

For information about special discounts for bulk purchases, please contact National Geographic Books Special Sales: specialsales@natgeo.com

For rights or permissions inquiries, please contact National Geographic Books Subsidiary Rights: bookrights@natgeo.com

Cover and interior design: Melissa Farris

Printed in the United States of America

16/xxx/1 [Product code, TK from Managing Ed. once printer is awarded]

For Liz

My buddy, my partner in adventure, my unwavering fan.
My rock, my fraggle, my favorite editor.

And, of course, my wife.

Contents

Introduction:
What Do You Expect?

IN 1978, THERE WAS A MINOR EPIDEMIC of Legionnaires' disease in Southern California. It was certainly not on the scale of the 1976 outbreak that had killed 34 people and introduced the disease to the world, but it made the news regularly. This acute bacterial pneumonia, named for its discovery at an American Legion meeting in Philadelphia, causes fever and intense coughing that occasionally brings up blood. Among the people watching those frightening broadcasts in California one spring evening were Sandy and Dee, a young couple who were practicing Christian Scientists. Their religion taught them that God created all his children in his own perfect image—and that with prayer, you could heal yourself, your family, and even people thousands of miles away. But to harness that ability, you needed the mental discipline to overlook what the rest of the world was telling you about human disease.

Their religion had served them well, until now. The news described a condition that sounded exactly like what was afflicting their one-and-a-half-year-old son, who had been looking pale and acting listless. The couple had been working with a Christian Science practitioner, or healer, who helped them pray for the child. But it didn't seem to be having any effect.

Dee, a lifelong Christian Scientist, had never doubted the power of her religion before. She had seen it heal dozens, maybe hundreds, of people and thought it was the very best care she could offer her son. Sandy, on the other hand, was a convert. A former professional baseball player, he had lost his spot on the Los Angeles Dodgers roster because of a painful shoulder injury that was miraculously cured six months later when he joined the Christian Science faith. In many ways, this made him even more devout than his wife was, even more sure that his religion was the best possible treatment for his son.

But fear is a powerful thing, especially when it comes to your children. Today we know that Legionnaires' disease is spread through the air—often through contaminated ventilation systems—and we have effective antibiotics for it. But in 1978, all anyone knew was that it struck without warning and was lethal in about 15 percent of adult cases. When Dee and Sandy saw the newscast explaining that a similar disease was killing scores of people in their area, they panicked and feared the worst. Christian Scientists believe that fear impedes one's ability to heal—and, sure enough, over course of the next day, the boy's condition worsened. One night it looked as though he was passing away in their arms. His face turned ashen, and his eyes rolled back in his head.

Dee, at her wits' end, considered for the first time going to a hospital—usually a last resort used only in the case of injuries like broken bones. For any of us, this might seem like the logical first step—something any loving parent would be obliged to do. For Dee, it was a frightening prospect, but she was too terrified to pray effectively and didn't know what else to do. Unless you have lived in a community of people who place their lives in the hands of their faith, it's hard to understand what it means to break from that guiding principle, to admit that what you've spent your life believing isn't working. It's even harder to understand what happened next.

Dee put her son down, went into the next room, and called her Christian Science healer yet again. Almost yelling, she gave the woman one last chance to affirm everything she believed in and had risked her son's life for. "I don't know if this religion works or not—but it damn well better work now!" she said, in a desperate and profound moment of doubt. "I'm losing my son!"

The practitioner began reassuring Dee, saying, "It doesn't matter whether this religion works or not. God loves your child." Over the next couple of minutes, everything changed for Dee. She let go of herself and put her trust in God. The world was transformed from a place where her son was dying and her community was helpless to save him into a world in which everything was perfect and God's love enveloped her family like a warm, comforting blanket.

Dee walked into the next room and saw what most people would describe as a miracle. Her child was sitting up, happy in his father's arms, his color returned, a smile on his face. Over the next few weeks, he seemed healed. The couple kept him isolated from other children while members of the church came to help care for the boy. He was happy, and nobody was worried about his having the disease anymore. Their religion had worked, and their faith had been rewarded.

● ● ●

I must have heard this story a thousand times growing up. You see, I was that dying child. For the first half of my life, the tenets of Christian Science were my only form of health care. I didn't visit a doctor's office until I was 18. Instead of popping pills or swallowing spoonfuls of bitter tonics, I used the Bible, the writings of Christian Science, and my own mind to heal myself.

Christian Science is an American religion founded in 1866. Its charismatic central founder, Mary Baker Eddy, claimed to have discovered the true meaning of Scripture: that all Christians have the ability to heal, just as Jesus did. Roughly speaking, Christian Scientists believe that all matter—your car, this book, or a shot of antibiotic—is superseded by a deeper reality based in the mind of God. In that reality, everyone and everything is perfect. Thus a healing comes through glimpsing a more perfect, truer version of yourself.

There are only a few hundred thousand Christian Scientists today, and very little research exists on their practices. One limited study from 1989, produced by the church's home office in Boston, attempted to quantify the healings that had taken place over the preceding 20 years. In that (admittedly not objective) paper, more than 2,000 Christian Scientists claim to have been spontaneously healed of medically diagnosed conditions across the spectrum: polio, bone cancer, ruptured appendixes, goiter, crossed eyes. There is even a 1966 story from South Africa in which a broken bone bulging out under the skin was healed over the course of a single day; this one strained credibility, even for an open-minded guy like me.

You name it, and Christian Scientists claim to have healed it. And they have a lot of company. The Internet is packed with cases of tumors eradicated by juice infusions, paralysis healed by the Holy Ghost, warts removed through hypnosis, and crippling pain erased in a single acupuncture session. Whether it's a revival meeting in the Florida Panhandle or a witch doctor in the jungles of eastern Mexico or some guy in Beijing who knows just the right way to rub your feet in order to relieve an upset stomach, mystical healing is all around us. When confronted with miracles or healings that we don't understand, most of us seem to respond with one of two reactions: "There must be forces out there beyond our comprehension" or the equally vague, but slightly more scientific "The mind is a powerful thing."

Both these statements are true. But neither is good enough for me, and shouldn't be for you either. In an era when we can beam real-time images of a working brain across the world—where a man missing his arm can use his mind to operate mechanical fingers to grip and even feel a plastic cup—it's time to expect a better answer.

All around us, permeating almost every aspect of our lives, is a profound mystery just waiting to be solved. It lives in daytime-TV stars hawking miracle vitamin pills; it lives in the mystical healing ability of someone burning incense while sticking needles in your forehead; and it lived in a small Southern California home where two people reached out to powers larger than themselves to save the life of their child. From homeopathy to shamanism, acupuncture to bizarre fad diets, people seem to have an innate ability to release pain, lose weight, and improve their lives by methods that just don't square with modern reason.

Or at least that's what I used to think.

In fact, there is a burgeoning field of science populated by an eclectic community of cutting-edge thinkers willing to look critically at what we loosely call mind/body healing. After spending the past few years immersed in their work, I have finally started to understand the healing practices I witnessed during my childhood. Scientists are casting light on the brain's unique power—for good or ill—to trick itself. These tricks can soothe us, make us sick, make us better, even save our lives. It's not a complete picture by any means. But it's the first we've had, and it offers a tempting opportunity to reshape 21st-century medicine as we know it.

But before I get into that, you might be wondering how a suburban faith healer ends up becoming a science writer. For the first half of my life, I never questioned the power of God to heal me. I could hear about someone who grew back a severed toe or spontaneously freed himself of AIDS and simply accept it. I believed that I had even heard the voice of God and that the entire world could heal itself with a single shift in thought. What happened? What could so shake a young man's certainty in his religion that he would leave it behind?

Rock climbing.

We all rebel a little when we hit puberty. But I didn't have the talent to join a rock band, the constitution for hard drugs, or the charm to sleep with girls. So I got into extreme sports. Pretty soon my Sunday mornings revolved less around church and more around adventures on the sides of cliffs. When I was 18, two friends and I decided to climb Lost Arrow Spire in Yosemite Valley. Imagine a sheer cliff, 2,000 feet high, with one of the world's tallest waterfalls on the left and nothing but empty space on the right. Now imagine a massive finger of granite leaning off the wall like a giant aggrieved splinter. That's Lost Arrow. The plan was to hike to the top of the cliff, rappel into the notch where the finger splits from the wall, climb the finger, and then cross back to where we started, via a rope spanning the 140-foot gap.

It's not a terribly difficult day's work for experienced climbers, and we figured we'd be done by mid-afternoon. What we did not figure was that a thunderstorm would roll in as we hung half a mile above the valley floor. I'd like to say it caught us off guard, but we knew one had been predicted for that afternoon. We just thought we were too fast to get caught in it. And that we were invincible.

The storm was a doozy. It came in hard, like an army of dump trucks dropped from B-2 bombers. The rain was mercifully thin, but the lightning was like nothing I had seen (or have seen in the 20 years since). It clapped and boomed and lit up the sky right above our heads. Vicious bolts of lightning, the heat of which momentarily parted the rain around us with surreal warmth, slammed two nearby peaks. The hair on my arms stood on end. I was sure I was about to die, draped in aluminum and clinging to the side of a giant granite lightning rod. All the while, Yosemite Falls roared to our left.

It was enough to make even a rebellious teenager put his trust in God.

So I tried. As my partners climbed the last 100 feet and I waited, hanging from a pair of metal rings bolted into a steep, blank wall, I prayed. I also cried, screamed, kicked uselessly at the wall, and did a fair amount of whimpering. But the praying is what I remember most. Because at that moment, after years of faith, I felt nothing. No "still small voice," no guiding presence, no flash of insight beyond a certainty that I was on my own.

When my turn came to climb, I felt a moment of peace and resolve, then clambered up that rock faster than I thought possible. As quickly as we could, we crossed the rope that spanned the gap between the spire and the safety of the main wall. Once we were all safely off the needle, the storm stopped.

Some might maintain that I was preserved by God's grace, even that I heard his voice in the storm itself; others, that the feeling of peace I felt before I went up the rope was really God giving me strength. But it wasn't. Many times, I have heard people say that God intervened in their lives in small ways: helping them find a parking space or encouraging them to talk to that cute boy at the other table. How did they know it was God? Because they felt his presence.

That day on Lost Arrow, I felt nothing but my own heartbeat and the knowledge that my fate was in my own hands (aided, perhaps, by a few laws relating to electrical fields). Just as others feel God and know he's there, I felt nothing and knew he wasn't. On that day, absence of evidence was evidence of absence. Whether it was God or just dumb luck that saved my life, I haven't felt anything like my childhood faith since. I attended a Christian Science college because it offered me a good scholarship, and I followed all its rules. But I was out: my exit card was punched. I was solidly dropped into the chaotic, often frightening material world of medicine, disease, and imperfection.

Yet, I've often thought about the healings I experienced and watched as a child. The relief that we in our community felt in times of sickness was real; it was palpable. Every Wednesday night, Christian Scientists have a special, less-scripted service than the Sunday version, in which people in the audience stand up and share their healings. These people aren't lying, and they aren't fooling themselves. Something else is happening. *Something* was giving me the power to heal myself as a child.

The nagging curiosity to understand that something compelled me to write this book. I'm not satisfied with explanations like "the mind is a powerful thing." What happened that day in 1978 with a toddler in Southern California? How can we explain the countless other instances of people being healed in ways that science has historically denied and disdained? Just as Copernicus pulled back a curtain of superstition and exposed a shiny new universe, brain scientists today are tugging at another curtain that promises answers to these questions.

• • •

One of the most important answers lies in the discovery that our brains are hardwired to trick themselves from time to time. The key to this ability lies in a single word: *expectation*. It's impossible to overstress just how important expectation is to the functioning of our brains. This is not just the feeling you have before the next season of *Game of Thrones* or when you are waiting to learn whether you got that job you wanted. Expectation is both the job description of the brain and its currency. It shapes how we think and move in the world around us. It dictates how we respond to music, how we experience food, how we communicate. Advertisers study expectation to shape their branding, economists study it to understand markets, and linguists study it to see how we understand what other people are saying. It is at work as you shift your feet and hands to hit a tennis ball and is there as you pause a second to inhale before taking that first sip of coffee in the morning. Think about it: Just putting one foot in front of the other requires expectation. In short, expectation is the way our brains process the world.

Your brain is wired to build expectations throughout your life over hours, years, or decades, then tries its best to turn those expectations into reality. Simply put, your brain doesn't want to be wrong—and in order for expectation to match reality, it's willing to bend a few rules or even cheat outright. As we shall learn, your brain's expectations are more powerful than we ever imagined. When those expectation clash with reality, more often than not, it's your stubborn brain that wins.

In 1996 the philosopher Daniel Dennett wrote, "A mind is fundamentally an anticipator, an expectation-generator." Our brains spend most of their time processing what they have already experienced in order to figure out what's about to happen. Imagine for a second that your brain failed to be an expectation-generator. You would essentially become a baby—everything would be novel and unpredictable. Nothing would make sense. Toss a ball up and it just keeps going. A dragon with the face of Harvey Keitel approaches you on the street and asks for directions. Reality-TV stars become more famous than actors with talent.

Expectation is just a system of shortcuts our brains have developed to get through life without stopping every five seconds to figure things out. You observe the world as best as you can, and then your brain fills in the gaps. But sometimes circumstances don't fit the model of the world that your brain has built. So rather than change its expectation, your brain will occasionally twist reality to bring your observations in line with your expectations. Therefore, if what you expect is negative, your mind will make things look (or feel) worse than they actually are. But if you expect the best—well, some pretty amazing things can happen in your body, as you'll see in the coming chapters. Somewhere in between this expectation and reality lies the mind's power to heal itself.

To access that power—that ability to use your brain to affect your body—you need a key that unlocks expectation. Many keys can tap into expectations and shape what we see around us every day. But the key that's been used by doctors, shamans, healers, and hucksters throughout the centuries is the power of suggestion. These two complementary ideas—*suggestion* and *expectation*—are at the heart of unlocking your internal medicine cabinet. They are also at the heart of my search for answers to my own childhood miracles.

The power of suggestion and expectation may be all around us—but tapping into it isn't easy, and it's not always clear when it happens. To do it, you have to completely shift your expectations to your advantage. In short, you need to make yourself suggestible. One way to do this is through storytelling. Nothing engages us quite as well as a good yarn, which can be very useful for suggestion. For instance, did you know that humans are just collections of molecules, made up of atoms, which themselves are nothing but energy? There is good energy and bad energy, and sometimes bad energy infiltrates parts of your body and makes you feel ill. But all you have to do is purify that energy—flush it out with good energy—and your symptoms will evaporate. Is this true? Not remotely. Still, for many people it sounds true. And that story—that suggestion—is enough to engage their expectation for healing.

Our uncanny ability to deceive ourselves holds startling implications for our health and well-being. Often what we call healings are tied to brain chemicals like opioid or dopamine. Some of these involve the placebo effect, which can coax remarkable reactions from areas of the brain involved with experiencing pain, nausea, Parkinson's, depression, irritable bowel syndrome, and other afflictions. It's perhaps the purest form of the brain's ability to alter reality, an undeniable neurochemical phenomenon. Another trick of the brain is placebo's alter ego, the nocebo effect, whereby our brain is fooled into *increasing* our discomfort and perhaps even creating disease from thin air. A third category is hypnosis, an odd little switch in the brain that gets activated and opens up a back door into our expectations. And the phenomenon of false memories tricks us into believing things that simply aren't so.

In these pages I will explore the hidden power, the history, and the science of human suggestibility. Along the way, we'll meet hypnotists, healers, magicians, and quacks. I'll personally be poked, prodded, electrocuted, burned, and even cursed. By the end, I hope to have revealed to you the secrets behind one of humanity's oldest stories—and the many ways they can affect your life.

Modern science is beginning to demonstrate that faith healing, miracle pills, and much of alternative medicine have one thing in common: you. Humans are deeply fallible creatures who build frameworks to explain the chaotic, confusing, and dangerous world that they live in. Those things that don't match their preconceptions are tossed aside or else twisted until they fit.

If this sounds like a depressing view of mankind, then you are in for a surprise. You see, that fallibility of mind—our suggestibility, if you will—is not a handicap; it can actually be one of our greatest assets. If used properly, our malleable minds can be twisted to our advantage, healing us and allowing us to live happier, healthier lives. But if used improperly, our suggestibility can be dangerous, even lethal.

Our brains have been subtly deceiving us since the dawn of time; we just haven't been able to see it until now. Today we are on the cusp of discovering the mysteries behind not just faith healing but also homeopathy, acupuncture, witchcraft, spells, herbal medicine, and many other treatments that have helped humanity, without our ever understanding why. What we are finding is not as clean or as simple as the heliocentric universe. But it is potentially just as important to the future of science as researchers probe the massive gulf between what we think and what actually is. The world, it turns out, is not what it seems. More important, it's not what we *expect* it to be. And in that fact lies unimaginable power.

This is the force that cured a small boy of Legionnaires' disease, that has been linked with Parkinson's disease and false memories, and that may be the greatest hope for those paralyzed by depression and chronic pain. Tracking this story has taken me through ancient and modern medicine to the brink of an exciting new precipice. Now close your eyes, forget what you think you know, and jump off with me.

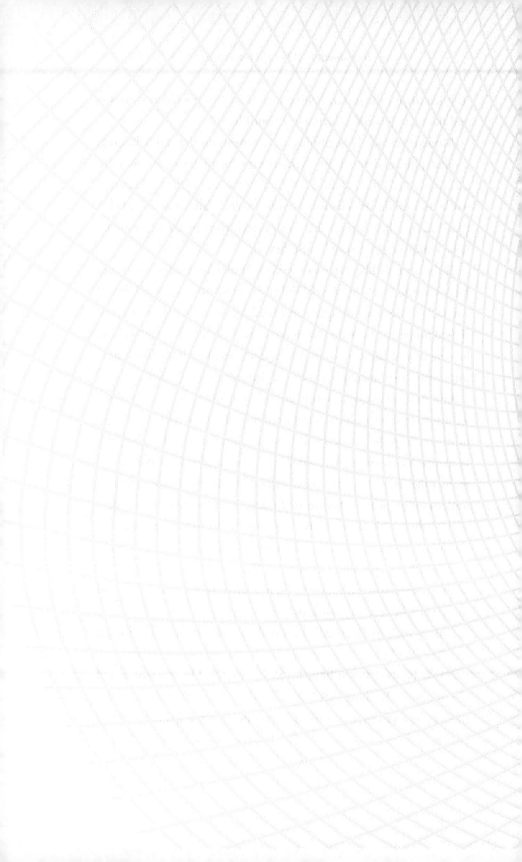

PART I

Inside *the* Placebo Effect

CHAPTER ONE

Placebos, Storytelling, *and the* Birth *of* Modern Medicine

The history of medicine is the history of the placebo effect.

—Arthur Shapiro and Louis Morris,
placebo researchers, 1978

THINK ABOUT THE LAST TIME you took a pain reliever for a headache. What did it look like? What size and shape was it? Was it white or pink? Which do you prefer? Do you need to see a name brand stamped on the side of it?

Now try to remember what it felt like when you swallowed it. As soon as you felt that pill go down, did you imagine molecules of the drug spreading cool, soothing relief into your head? Did you feel better immediately? If you did, that's strange because most painkillers take about 15 to 20 minutes to kick in. That feeling of immediate relief many people experience is the placebo effect—perhaps the purest form of suggestion and expectation. From the Latin for "I shall please," *placebo* traditionally refers to anything inert that has an effect on a patient, usually lasting less than a day but sometimes longer: a sugar pill, a saline injection, or sham surgery, often mixed with a little smoke and mirrors. In other words, nothing. But in the world of expectation, sometimes nothing is more powerful than something—if it's wrapped in the right packaging.

That packaging is different for everybody. What allows a placebo to work is something scientists are still trying to understand. It's a combination of psychology, chemistry, and genetics, aided by the power of storytelling. And it all depends on how that placebo is presented. In the case of the headache pill, it's wrapped in the package of Western medicine: something you've come to trust will bring relief. But there are hundreds of other ways to tap into placebos, as scientists are still discovering today.

Contrary to popular wisdom, placebos are not tricks or sleight of hand for the gullible or weak-minded—and they're not always temporary. In fact, they are measurable, tangible brain events. Far from something to be scorned, the placebo effect is actually the cornerstone of the modern pharmaceutical industry and, for some people, a ticket to better health and well-being. Let me give you an example of what I mean.

In 2003, Natalie Grams was a young medical student working in a hospital in Heidelberg, Germany. Her view of medicine was in keeping with that of any physician: Disease is the result of physical problems in the body; understand its mechanisms, correctly diagnose the symptoms, administer the right treatment, and you can beat it. She treated her patients as many doctors do, going from one symptom to the next, prescribing this or that drug after a few minutes of gathering data.

Then one day she took a literal turn in the road that changed everything. She was driving near her home when a car coming the opposite way drifted into her lane. She had to veer off the road to avoid a head-on collision. Her car spun hard and then rolled several times down a slope into the woods. Miraculously, Grams walked away from the wreck without any physical injuries beyond a little whiplash. But not long afterward, she started having disabling panic attacks that made her feel like she was suffocating. At first they were a nuisance; then they became a genuine concern. After she experienced an attack while at work in the operating room, she realized that they were debilitating for her and perhaps lethal for her patients. She consulted multiple doctors who checked her for lung problems, infections, and half a dozen other potential triggers. She tried psychiatry and took anti-anxiety medication, but nothing helped. Finally, she went to a homeopath.

Homeopathy was created in Germany at the beginning of the 19th century by a young doctor named Samuel Hahnemann. A keen observer of human nature, he was disgusted by the practices he observed in medicine at the time, especially bloodletting. He saw physicians of his era doing more harm than good, and believed the best medicine was often bed rest and a good diet. Fascinated by various types of remedies, he experimented on himself and noticed that a healthy person who takes quinine—used to treat malaria—gets malaria-like symptoms. What if that very similarity between illness and treatment was what led to healing? Maybe physicians needed to find a cure that came in a package similar to the disease itself. *"Similia similibus curantur,"* he said: Like cures like. It was a powerful notion that seemed intuitively correct. Furthermore, Hahnemann hypothesized that it wasn't the chemical itself that brought relief but the *essence* of that chemical. Thus, you could dilute the cure with water until the compound was nonexistent, and the water would convey that essence of cure to the patient.

"I did not believe in it," Grams told me. "I had had no contact with this so-called medicine before. And I was completely surprised at how much time [the homeopath] had, how much she looked at me as a person and not just symptoms. I thought, 'This is the missing part of my medical life.' "

Grams's homeopath recommended belladonna, or deadly nightshade, a poisonous bush used throughout history for political assassination. Naturally, she wouldn't get a pure dose but one that had been diluted down to one part for every novemdecillion (that's a one with 60 zeroes after it) parts water. In other words, every molecule of nightshade had long since been purged from the liquid and all that was left was water.

Now, there is no scientific reason why deadly nightshade, let alone highly diluted deadly nightshade, should have helped Grams's panic disorder when prescription drugs had failed. But it did: Her symptoms dissipated. She was floored. There must, she reasoned, be some unseen, unstudied mechanism behind this amazing healing art that science had ignored. Against warnings from her colleagues, who said it would sabotage her medical career, she decided to become a homeopath herself. In seven years she was practicing homeopathy, and three years later she opened her own practice.

Her prescriptions targeted not the symptoms of her patients but the way they described them. A pain in the chest that made patients say they felt "trapped" or "compressed" would be treated totally differently from one that they described as feeling like heat, for example. One of Grams's patients during this time was so paralyzed by depression that she couldn't leave her house. She had tried years of psychotherapy and medications but had become a deeply depressed shut-in and an alcoholic. After talking to her about her condition for hours, Grams found that the woman traced her sadness to one frigid night in her childhood, when she and her parents had fled the Nazis. Her symptoms, interestingly, were much worse during the cold German winters.

Treating like with like, Grams hit upon a prescription that reflected the power of that cold night decades before: regular doses of melted snow. In other words, water. Amazingly, after a few sessions, the treatment started to work. The woman improved, gave up drinking, and eventually began traveling to nearby towns to visit friends. Whenever she felt an attack of depression or anxiety coming on, she reached for a vial of melted snow.

Grams's practice grew until she was making far more as a homeopath than she had as a doctor. So she decided to write a book about the power of homeopathy, aimed at audiences like her old colleagues—and her former self—who had been skeptical of it. She would use empirical evidence to show that homeopathy was effective and thus prove Hahnemann's philosophy.

But the more she dug into the scientific literature, the more she learned that the homeopathic treatments she had been administering showed zero merit in careful scientific tests. The few studies that claimed small successes generally had a tiny group of test subjects, included statistical biases, or involved less aggressive dilutions than those used in normal homeopathic practice (meaning they contained more of the active ingredient). Homeopaths make the argument that a mysterious active ingredient is driving all this, but decades of searching haven't turned up anything. One skeptic organization called 10:23 even demonstrated this by drinking entire bottles of the stuff in a publicity stunt meant to show that you can't overdose on homeopathic remedies. The logic being, how can there be an active ingredient if it is impossible to overdose? After hundreds of trials, most scientists have come to the conclusion that homeopathic remedies are actually placebos.

What's going on here? Homeopathy improved the health of Grams, her patients, and hundreds of thousands of other people and is one of the most popular forms of alternative medicine in existence. How does it work so well if it's not real? How can it be the placebo effect when Grams herself didn't even believe in homeopathy when she started it?

In essence, homeopathic treatments create suggestion through expert storytelling—a key that fits the magic lock in our brains' expectations. Recall how much time Grams's homeopath spent talking to her and, in turn, how much time Grams spent trying to understand her patients' stories. This was not therapy, which is meant to help patients confront or understand or overcome their problems. We can't say for sure whether her patient's debilitating depression can be traced to that terrifying night decades earlier. But that's not the point. The suggestion that it might be the cause resonated deeply with her, and that was enough. The stories we are told—and those we tell ourselves—shape our vision of the world. Grams expertly took a story that resonated with her patient and redirected it to help her escape the crippling fear that was trapping her in her home.

In the course of the year that Grams spent writing her book, however, it dawned on her that she might be a fraud. "It was a very hard year," she says. "I had many sleepless nights and a lot of tears. I was afraid at one point. I knew that I was treating patients who had really serious problems like cancer, like depression, like chronic pain."

She overcame her heartbreak and published her book anyway. Instead of exonerating homeopathy, the book condemned it as little more than a compelling story delivered by attentive, skilled caregivers. The day it was published, she closed her practice and turned her back on homeopathy forever. Today she is focusing on being a mother and working to get homeopathy curricula removed from German universities and medical practice.

• • •

Placebos certainly didn't start with Grams or even Hahnemann. Plato was in favor of occasionally fibbing to fool patients into having a response to dubious remedies. Hippocrates, a fellow Greek who lived around the same time, also understood the power of the body to heal itself but opposed such mind games. He spent his life upending the pageantry of shamans who treated patients through appeals to the gods, observing that sometimes doing nothing is preferable to quack treatment. One of Hippocrates' two lasting contributions to medicine was the idea that quiet rest is the first step to good treatment (summarized by the famous mantra "do no harm," which was coined 2,000 years later) and is itself a kind of placebo.1

Since then, humans have invented legions of bizarre treatments that we know today to be placebos: Syphilis catheters, partridge brains, urine baths, bird poop, baby poop, the blood of a black chicken, spiders, human fat, mercury, and good old bloodletting are just a few. As more people turned from mysticism to science, however, it became clear that not everything the local snake oil salesman was peddling was worth the price. (Not counting snake oil itself, which I've found to be a great painkiller when mixed with hard rice wine in Vietnamese dive bars.)

Eventually, people began casting about for a way to separate the good remedies from the bad. Around 1025, the legendary Persian doctor and mathematician Avicenna wrote his *Canon of Medicine*, which lays out parameters for clinical tests of new drugs that are surprisingly in sync with modern standards. Among other rules, he said that the drugs being tested must be pure (with no additives that might confuse matters), must work consistently, and must work on people—not just on horses and lions. Today's laboratory experiments follow similar rules—except we substitute mice for lions. Most

---

1 His other lasting contribution was a system of medicine based on the four humors—or bodily fluids. It was a huge step forward from the superstitious god-based medicine of the time because it said that disease starts in the body and not on Mount Olympus. Everything else about it was wrong, however, and it led to a thousand years of superstitious, humor-based medicine.

29

important, three of his seven rules warn against "accidental cures." Though he didn't use the word "placebo," it's clear that even then he was worried that drugs without any active ingredients might slip into use.

The man who often gets credit for conducting the first true "clinical" trial, comparing one remedy with another, is the Scottish physician James Lind. In 1747, he discovered that citrus fruits like oranges and limes are useful for curing scurvy, an ailment caused by a lack of vitamin C in the diet. He did this with a simple side-by-side test involving giving sick sailors one of the following: citrus fruit, vinegar, cider, sulfuric acid, seawater, or a spice cocktail of his own invention. (It should be noted that, strictly speaking, none of these was technically a placebo at the time, since all were already rumored to cure scurvy.) After a couple of days, only the citrus-eaters were ready for duty. Unfortunately for British gums, the discovery was mostly ignored at first. But it eventually got picked up by a few enterprising captains and later became so popular that many British sailors walked around with limes in their mouths, resulting in the nickname limeys.[2]

Twenty-five years later, a bizarre health fad created an opportunity for a truly placebo-controlled trial. Franz Mesmer, a highly intelligent, charismatic doctor, was fascinated by the motions of the planets and the relationship they might have on the human body. He had been inspired by a small-town country priest named Johann Joseph Gassner, who made a name for himself doing exorcisms using nothing but the sound of his commanding voice. Gassner wrote numerous treatises on his technique, which we now recognize as a form of hypnotism

---

2 As for Lind, in 1753 he discovered that shaving and bathing sailors from time to time and washing their bedsheets eradicates typhus fever, which is spread by fleas and lice. This surely helped the British defeat the French in the Napoleonic Wars. When Lind died, he had achieved the high honor of Knight Commander of the Order of the Bath—apparently awarded without a trace of irony.

(although he attributed it to the voice of God working through his spoken word). No one had ever seen anything like it, and Mesmer was understandably blown away.

Mesmer didn't believe in demons and wasn't particularly religious, so he had a tough time swallowing Gassner's interpretations of his power. But when he noticed that the priest used a metal crucifix during his fantastic exorcisms, a light went on. It wasn't superstition or religion; it was science. Mesmer concluded that Gassner's ability to heal people was based not on his voice or the power of God, but on *magnetism* unwittingly channeled through his metal crucifixes. He extrapolated that this was the key to all the objects in the universe, including the human body. Mesmer observed that, like the tides in the sea and the planets in the sky, the human body was awash in magnetism. He reasoned that the same forces that drew metal objects together created a sort of invisible "universally spread fluid" that swirls around us (kind of like the Force from *Star Wars*). He believed that certain people (let's call them Jedi) could manipulate this fluid with their minds, as a conductor directs a symphony, and even heal afflictions. He called this force animal magnetism (not to be confused with the modern, sexy meaning of this term).

Never mind that neither the tides nor planetary orbits are controlled by magnetism—they're controlled by the more powerful and confusing force of gravity. Never mind that the human body isn't remotely magnetic and that there's no reason why magnets would obey the human mind. As with homeopathy, magnetism is the kind of idea that made sense at a visceral level. *Yeah, magnets—that's what it's all about!* It was similar to the way people talk about quantum physics today: a complicated, ill-understood phenomenon that seems important, but one that people just can't wrap their heads around. So they did the next best thing: They found a few metaphors and ran with it.

Mesmer's idea was simple. Assuming that magnet juice was everywhere and that it obeyed his will, he could use that power to magnetize, say, a vat of water so that it had the power to heal people who touched it. Or, better yet, the power to heal people who touched things that had touched it. Or, you know, just got near it. Looking at it today, it was no more accurate than Gassner's ideas about demons. But as with the priest's, Mesmer's techniques worked..

Of course, Mesmer had tapped into not magnetism but the placebo effect. Yes, our bodies do exert a weak electromagnetic force. And yes, water—including the water in our bodies—can be magnetized, meaning that all the molecules can be arranged in the same direction, the positive ends facing one way and the negative ends facing the other. All it takes is a magnetic field about 3,400 times stronger than your average handheld magnet. And about 16 *trillion* times stronger than the magnetism in the human body.

But Mesmer and his acolytes believed they could harness the power of magnet juice using their minds alone. And it worked. Want to know why? Because Mesmer was a master of theatrics. First of all, he cut an impressive figure, wearing a leather shirt lined with silk and hung with magnets that he said kept his magnetic fluid from escaping. He was charismatic, intelligent, and utterly convincing. In his salon he played strange music and turned the lights down low. In the middle of the room was a cauldron of magnetized water. People would sit and reverently hold iron rods submerged in the water. With their other hands they held the fingers of the person next to them or a circular rope to pass the magnetism from one person to the next.

After the treatment was concluded, participants claimed to be cured of all manner of ailments: psychological maladies, chronic pain, even blindness. When people were exposed to Mesmer's power—or even to the water that he had "treated"—they would fall into convulsions. These reportedly lasted for hours, sometimes causing the victim—sorry, patient—to spit up blood and "murky expectoration" (apparently the Victorian word for "loogie"). Mesmer even built a special padded room for particularly violent patients to use while they convulsed. One observer at the time wrote, "Because of these constant effects, one cannot help but acknowledge the presence of a great power which moves & controls patients, & which resides in the magnetizer."

Mesmer was a master of two classic mechanisms of a placebo. First, there was his ability for storytelling. To harness expectation, you need a convincing story—one so seamless and engaging that it leaves no room for doubt. Whether through magnets, or magically treated water, or a black chicken's blood, suggestibility demands a tale that resonates with the individual patient. Second, he had tapped into the "theater of medicine." Like any convincing performance, the medical theater requires its trappings to be convincing. Even modern medicine relies on costumes (white coats), props (a stethoscope around the neck), and set design (the clean white walls of an office adorned with a schematic of the human body). Although he may not have realized it, Mesmer had both the story and the theater in which to present it.

Mesmer founded a school in Vienna, but he eventually found his way to France and the court of King Louis XVI. Eighteenth-century Paris was the cultural and economic center of Europe and the center of the universe for aspiring intellects like Mesmer. The city went wild for this charming foreigner; his clinic was booked weeks in advance. (Originally he'd magnetized people individually, but ultimately he had to switch to the vats of magnetized water to keep up with demand.) His devotees included Amadeus Mozart (who later seemed to have lost some respect for the doctor, whom he satirized in *Così Fan Tutte*), as well as the French queen Marie Antoinette. At first the king seemed content to allow Mesmer to go about his business, and even supported him for a while. But in 1784 he became suspicious and set up a commission to investigate Monsieur Mesmer's claims.

The commission was a Who's Who of French scholarship, including Antoine Lavoisier (often called the father of modern chemistry), Joseph-Ignace Guillotin (who inspired the device later used to cut off Lavoisier's and Marie Antoinette's heads), and, I kid you not, Benjamin Franklin. In one of those wonderful historical moments that seem scripted by Hollywood, Franklin happened to be in town acting as the first ambassador to France from the newly formed United States of America.

Interestingly, Franklin and company chose to focus their investigation on Charles d'Eslon, one of Mesmer's most devoted students and the fellow who had laid out the theory of animal magnetism before the French Faculty of Medicine a few years before, in 1780. (Why they didn't target Mesmer himself seems a bit unclear. I presume it was political. One had to be careful when attacking the reputation of a man with so many fans in the French aristocracy.) The commission descended upon poor d'Eslon like parrots on a cracker convention. They started with a relatively simple question: Does animal magnetism even exist? Or, as they put it, significantly less simply: "Animal magnetism may well exist without being useful but it cannot be useful if it does not exist." (I'd argue that plenty of things that don't exist are useful, such as homeopathic remedies and Santa Claus.)

The team attacked the problem methodically, one piece at a time. They found that animal magnetism couldn't be detected by sight, sound, smell, or taste (though they failed to mention how they verified that last one). Nor, oddly enough, could it be detected with magnets. In fact, very few people could sense it at all. Two hundred and fifty years later, you can almost hear their frustration. "Patients then display a variety of reactions depending on the different states they find themselves in. Some are calm, quiet, & feel nothing; others cough, spit, feel slight pain, a warmth either localized or all over, & perspire; others are agitated & tormented by convulsions."

Right away, the commission seemed skeptical of these fits. At the time, most physicians were little more than witch doctors themselves, experimenting with healing techniques as they went, and snake oil salesmen were rampant on both sides of the Atlantic. A few still even used Hippocrates' medicine based on humors. But the notion of the mind's healing power was well understood; indeed, Franklin's friend and colleague Thomas Jefferson would occasionally take inert pills made of bread to treat minor illnesses.

So the team gathered up a group of test subjects the same way I assume most gentleman scientists did in those days—from their household staffs. Out of 11 volunteers, they found one, a "doorkeeper" (or doorwoman), who claimed she could sense animal magnetism on her skin (when a hand was moved across her, she felt a sense of heat, like a flame). Many of Mesmer's clients were women, causing the scientists to wonder in a secret letter to the king whether the response might be related to some kind of heightened "female sensitivity."

It was a sexist assumption that has followed placebos to this very day, but in one way they may have had a point. Eighteenth-century France was surely an oppressively dull place for the idle rich, especially women. Then along came Mesmer, whose sessions were exciting, intellectually engaging, and oddly social. (As we will see in later chapters, suggestibility relies partially on belief and good storytelling but receives a boost from the power of social pressure.) The commission quickly realized that if they wanted to get to the truth, they needed to get d'Eslon away from his home turf. So they invited him and a few of his favorite clients to Franklin's estate to conduct a series of tests.

First, they asked d'Eslon to magnetize a tree in an orchard. Then, they asked one of his patients to guess which one it was. Sure enough, the man began to sweat, got headaches, and eventually passed out when he got close to one of the trees. Just not the right tree. In fact, his fits became worse as he moved farther away from the tree that d'Eslon had focused on. The mesmerist explained that this was because all trees, being living organisms, are somewhat magnetized and that this man was so sensitive even an unaugmented tree could make him pass out.

They conducted 16 of these tests over the next few weeks. My favorite involved a woman who claimed to be sensitive to magnetized water. Now, just to be clear, the water was not actually magnetized, any more than the tree was. Water molecules are indeed lopsided (with all the oxygen on one side) and can thus theoretically respond to magnets. However, to actually move them in any direction, they would need to wait a couple of centuries for much more powerful magnets, and the effect would last only a fraction of a second. And it wouldn't affect a person's health.

But never mind. The commission asked d'Eslon to magnetize a glass of water. Then they brought a different, identical glass of water to the woman. Immediately sensing the magical power of magnetization, she fainted on the spot. When she came to, the gentlemen soothed her and brought her a glass of water to revive her. That glass, as you might have guessed, was filled with the "magnetized" water. She drank it gratefully and felt much better.

Not surprisingly, the commission came out against Mesmer and d'Eslon, proclaiming, "No doubt the imagination of patients often has an influence upon the cure of their maladies . . . It is a well-known adage that in medicine faith saves; this faith is the product of the imagination."

The report was a crushing blow to Mesmer, exposing him as a fraud (though maybe a well-meaning one). He disappeared from high society not long after and lived his remaining days in the countryside. I doubt that Benjamin Franklin thought much about the project afterward; it was a mere postscript to a staggeringly important scientific career. But his exercise in reason on behalf of a doomed French king began exposing a long-buried truth that would someday shake the foundation of modern medicine to its core.

● ● ●

It took a few years for the word "placebo" to be coined, but Mesmer clearly understood the concept and in some ways, he had foreseen modern brain science as well. You see, the human brain is adept at finding patterns. We use those patterns to look for danger, spot food, and make predictions about what's about to happen. Much of this pattern spotting and expectation generating is crucial for the placebo response but doesn't happen on a conscious level. Take one of the most primal placebo triggers, classical conditioning. Conditioning, as you may remember from high school, is what Pavlov did to make his dog drool. Ring a bell, give food. Ring a bell, give food. Do that enough times and the dog will drool whenever you ring a bell, regardless of food. Pavlov was tapping into the dog's expectation systems. It had been *conditioned* to expect food when it heard the bell.

Over the years, scientists have used classical conditioning to tap into all kinds of placebo responses from unwitting subjects. In the 1970s, they programmed rats to shut off their immune response through the power of conditioning and expectation by pairing an immunosuppressant with a sweet drink. Every time the rat took the drink, it also got a drug called cyclosporin A, which blocks immune response (it's often used in transplant surgery to keep the new body from rejecting the organ). After a while, the scientists could administer the drink by itself and the rats' immune system would deactivate their immune response, or T cells, just as if they had been given the drug.

Similar experiments have shown that the same tricks could manipulate a slew of other immune system triggers in rats, including lymphocytes, leucocytes, and natural killer cells—all of which play a role in how our bodies respond to infectious disease. Most important, researchers have shown that the same trick can work on people. Obviously, if I told you to adjust your lymphocytes (white blood cells in your lymphatic system) down by 30 percent right now, you wouldn't be able to do it. But if I mixed a lymphocyte-lowering drug into a sweet-flavored drink and gave it to you on multiple occasions, and then just started giving you the drink without the drug, your body might do it on its own.

That's because your body has been conditioned to the drug, and when it doesn't get it, it simply acts as if it had. Think about the last time an ailment sent you to the doctor's office. Did you feel as bad in the examining room as you had at home or in the car? Studies suggest that you probably didn't. Whether through a sudden rush of lymphocytes or just self-delusion, we generally report feeling better as soon as we feel we're under the care of the doctor. Because we are conditioned to expect to feel better.

This is tied directly to the theater of medicine. The trappings of healing—the "story"—immediately put us in the frame of mind that we are receiving treatment and build our confidence in it. Just like Mesmer, a doctor can unconsciously trigger a placebo: a kindly hand on your shoulder, eye contact, a sense of confidence and authority. Then there are all the accoutrements, such as the white coat, the fancy tools, the jars of Q-tips and gauze. All of it communicates to our subconscious that it's time to feel better.

You might be wondering whether learning about this might stop it from working for you in the future. Are you eating from the forbidden fruit of knowledge, so that the next time you pop an Advil, you won't feel anything until it kicks in? Never fear. Classical conditioning happens largely on an unconscious level. You can no more prevent your placebo response than Pavlov's puppy can keep from drooling. This has even been shown in the laboratory. A team of Harvard researchers conducted an experiment in which they told subjects they were getting placebos—and the subjects still felt relief.

Why? In part because they, like most of us, had been conditioned their whole lives to believe that when you take a pill, you feel better. And part of that conditioning comes from looking around the room, experiencing the patterns of the theater of medicine you've come to recognize—the doctor, the lab coat, even the smell of disinfectant—and responding just like the drooling dog. This theater plays out in thousands of ways. For instance, depression patients respond better to yellow placebo pills than to blue ones. Bigger ones work better than smaller ones, but only to a certain point (at which the pill is just too big to believe, I suppose). Fake injections work better than fake pills. And if you're French, suppositories work better than either. Take a quiet moment to ponder the significance of that.

As a child, I was conditioned to respond to the distinctive and powerful voice of my Christian Science practitioner. These practitioners—combination therapists-friends-teachers—are people you call on when you need help or feel sick and can be amazing. I remember vividly the power of my practitioner's voice. Her name was Lamiece, and I truly believed she could work miracles. She had cured everything from colds to cancer. Word was that she had even cured AIDS once—the virus simply left the man's body. For a suggestible young kid, having a woman like that on your side meant having some serious firepower. My mother told me (in a way that said "there's a bigger story here that you are not old enough to hear") that Lamiece had seen more than her share of life's challenges; this gave her the mysterious air of a combat veteran. Her dark eyes could stare right into your soul, and then there was that voice. I'd call her up with a sniffle or a fever, and on the other end a voice that was a perfect cross between that of Glinda the Good Witch and the Oracle in *The Matrix* would pick up. Immediately I would feel better. I can still hear her perfectly graveled alto on the other end of the phone—maternal, weathered, and as tough as nails—telling me that everything was going to be OK and that God loved me. To this day, it's the most comforting voice I can imagine.

• • •

While Mesmer might have mastered the theater of healing and his persecutors dabbled in placebo controls, it took another 150 years before scientists really looked at the placebo effect carefully. As with most breakthroughs in science, there was no single eureka moment in the discovery of the placebo effect. But most say the modern concept of placebos began with Henry Beecher, a doctor on the North African and Italian fronts in World War II. Beecher's interest in placebos was inspired largely by the intensity of what he witnessed in that war. Imagine for a moment being a soldier in North Africa whose body has been riddled with shrapnel. There is the initial shock and confusion, the momentary notion that the explosive has missed you, and the attempt to get up. Then the realization that you're covered in blood and that your unit is working desperately to stanch the wounds and drag you to safety. For that first hour, adrenaline and fear cover the pain.

But then comes the 10-hour drive down brutally bumpy roads to the field hospital. Your buddies and the field medic are acting oddly, and you could swear there's something on the stretcher poking you under your back. By the time you get to the hospital, you are dying of thirst. Around you are the sounds of people screaming, one of them begging to die. And that blasted joint on the stretcher is still sticking in your back. A doctor asks if you want any morphine. *Oh, Jesus, I'm not that bad off,* you think; morphine is for people on their deathbed, you tell him. No, just give me some more water. The doctor gives you a shot of something, and you wince at the pain of the injection. Then he turns you over and exposes what he will later describe as an ax-like wound on your back from the shrapnel.

This was just one of the experiences Beecher witnessed and puzzled over. How could that man wince at the injection yet not notice the gaping wound in his back? It must have been a surreal experience for a genteel Midwesterner on leave from a cushy job at Harvard. When he joined the war effort, he wasn't a bright-eyed kid looking for a fight; he was a middle-age Ivy League anesthesiologist working for the government, studying the effects of morphine and other drugs on a battlefield. At first, his letters and reports were bursting with excitement about the scientific secrets he was about to uncover. But as the war continued, his reports revealed more and more frustration. He commented on the lack of drugs, equipment, and manpower. And equipment that did arrive was either the wrong size or was missing components. Eventually he left his post with the War Department and went straight into the Army as a doctor. But he was first and foremost a scientist. As the war went on, he collected all manner of data—how long it took a patient to get to care, what drugs were given, and most important, whether they even wanted any.

It was this last question that seems to have stuck with him the most. Here were young men with grisly wounds who hadn't seen any painkillers in hours, yet they seemed relatively unimpaired. In one paper examining 215 patients with "major wounds," he noted that 40 of the 50 patients with "penetrating wounds of the thorax" declined painkillers. A similar ratio of people with head wounds and "extensive soft-tissue wounds" did as well. He'd seen terrible injuries in civilian hospitals after accidents, and the patients begged for drugs. Why should a soldier be immune to pain? And how could that same soldier turn around and complain "bitterly" about the pain of a tiny needle? What separated those who felt pain from those who didn't? As the war was ending, he mused: "Strong emotion can block pain. That is common experience. In this connection, it is important to consider the position of the soldier: his wound suddenly releases him from an exceedingly dangerous environment, one filled with fatigue, discomfort, anxiety, fear, and real danger of death, and gives him a ticket to the safety of the hospital. His troubles are over—or he thinks they are."

On the other hand, a civilian's accident marks the beginning of disaster for him. It is impossible to say whether this produces an increased awareness of his pain and increased suffering; possibly it does. Beecher also noticed that many of his soldier-patients found relief after taking sulfonamide pills, made for preventing fevers, which are antibiotics and have nothing to do with pain. "Such pain," he wrote, "must have been due to suggestion."

Beecher puzzled over these questions for the rest of his career. And he wasn't the only one who noticed that pain could be relative. The statistician and Yale professor E. Morton Jellinek was among the first to quantify the placebo effect, though accidentally. In 1946, Jellinek was asked by representatives for a manufacturer—he didn't say which—to test a mysterious headache drug ("drug A") containing ingredients a, b, and c. The b ingredient was in short supply after the war, and the company was hoping to just leave it out for a while. Naturally they wanted to know if their drug would still work without that ingredient.

So Jellinek, who specialized in teasing out conclusions from complex data, created a blind trial with 199 patients in four groups using physically identical pills. One pill had all three ingredients; one had just a and b; another had just a and c; and the last was a lactate placebo. (Sugar was originally the placebo of choice, but because sugar isn't truly inert, modern placebo pills tend to be made of ingredients like corn oil or lactose. They're not totally inert but probably as close as it gets.) Each person who suffered regular headaches took a pill whenever one came on and wrote down whether it worked. Every two weeks they switched to the next pill, so that after eight weeks everyone had tried every pill. Jellinek then compiled all the data and started calculating.

But he quickly ran into a problem. A full 120 of the 199 people seemed to do just as well on the placebo as on any of the other drugs. Moreover, all the active pills seemed equally effective (meaning the company didn't need ingredient b). But then Jellinek examined the 79 people who *didn't* respond to the placebo. Among this sample, the pills with all the ingredients were the most effective, followed by the ones missing ingredient c. Last were the ones missing ingredient b. In other words, he wrote, yes, they did need ingredient b in their drug. In fact, for 40 percent of them, it was the only part of the pill they couldn't afford to lose. What he didn't say, however, was that they could also just ditch ingredients a, b, *and* c—give people a placebo—and 60 percent of their customers would never even notice.

Jellinek's study foreshadowed two placebo trends over the next 50 years. First, it foresaw a revolutionary new era for evaluating medicine. Soon drugs would have to be

1. randomized (distributed to patients randomly),
2. double-blind (neither patients nor doctors would know who got what), and
3. placebo-controlled (shown to be more effective than a placebo).

Second, it also heralded a new tendency to discredit people who respond to placebos. In his final report, Jellinek accurately realized that the difference between those who responded to the placebo and those who didn't had something to do with the nature of the people with the headaches. But rather than investigate why this was, he seemed to blame the subjects themselves. The people who responded only to the drug, he wrote, were a "pure culture of physiological headaches not accessible to suggestion." The other 120 subjects must have had milder "psychogenic headaches" coupled with a "tendency toward suggestibility."

Seen through a 1946 lens, a "tendency toward suggestibility" looks a lot like "sucker." After a truly ingenious study, Jellinek examined the data and could not fathom why so many of his subjects seemed to repeatedly get better on lactate pills.

Neither could almost all those who came after him. They were interested only in the people who responded to a drug, not in the ones who got better with a placebo. Thus, for more than 30 years, the placebo effect was barely studied, except by a few oddball scientists who risked being labeled as nutty or fringe. Although it wasn't interesting in itself to most scientists, the placebo effect did present a sizable problem. With so many people responding to placebos, how could pharmaceutical companies know whether it was their drugs or the *suggestion* of their drugs that healed people?

In 1955, after years of contemplating these issues, Henry Beecher wrote a breakthrough paper called "The Powerful Placebo," which assembled stories like Jellinek's. By this time, Beecher had become a major figure in anesthesiology because of his work during World War II, and this was the first important paper to address placebos directly. He estimated that about 30 percent of patients across all of medicine have placebo responses to any given drug. When one of the nation's leading pain experts says that a third of the people who take pain drugs might be imagining their relief, it gets noticed.[3]

---

3 It's worth mentioning that at the same time that Beecher was doing his groundbreaking work on placebos, many say he also dabbled heavily in interrogation and torture research. Historian Alfred McCoy at the University of Wisconsin believes he was a key player in the U.S. effort to convert psychotropic drugs like mescaline and LSD into a truth serum, much of which was inspired by Nazi scientists. Many servicemen suffered lifelong psychological problems after volunteering for such experiments.

The discovery in the 1950s of some invisible force making fake medicines appear to work was about as jarring as a magnitude 9 earthquake in a china shop—and only marginally less welcome. People started wondering whether drugs should be measured against the effect of placebo pills before being released to the public. Such placebo-controlled trials had been used occasionally by scientists since the turn of the century, but usually they were conducted for curiosity's sake, as with Jellinek's headache drug, and not as any kind of official litmus test. At the time, the only thing a drugmaker had to do to certify a product was to prove that it wouldn't kill patients. Or, you know, not too many patients.

But Beecher and an acolyte, Johns Hopkins pharmacology professor Lou Lasagna (his real name, I swear), were pushing for drugs to be both safe *and* effective. Soon they were joined by Tennessee senator Estes Kefauver (also his real name), who took up the cause in 1959 and started crusading for mandatory clinical drug trials. Kefauver held numerous Senate hearings under the Antitrust and Monopoly Subcommittee, where he badgered drug company representatives for alleged price fixing and the high costs of drugs that might not even work. The pharmaceutical industry struck back with dual arguments that boiled down to: 1) "Hey, do you know someone else who can make this stuff?" and 2) "If it wasn't working, people wouldn't be getting better, would they?" To which Kefauver would reply: If it works so well, why not prove it? To which the pharma people would respond, "Why test what we know works?" And around and around.

Lasagna had a dogged but not very effective advocate in the senator. Kefauver had made so many enemies over the years that Lyndon Johnson once called him the most hated man in Congress. (A few years before, along with Johnson, he had been among the few southern congressmen who refused to sign the Southern Manifesto, decrying school integration. Although courageous and deeply moral, this did not make him popular.) After a few years it became clear that nothing would come of the hearings because conservatives hated Kefauver and liberals didn't want to antagonize pharmaceutical companies while President Kennedy was pushing for the passage of Medicaid. Perhaps nothing would have changed had it not been for the thalidomide disaster of 1961.

Thalidomide was a European drug prescribed to alleviate the symptoms of morning sickness in pregnant women. Today it's known as the greatest catastrophe in the history of the pharmaceutical industry. You see, no one had bothered to find out whether this morning-sickness drug was safe for the unborn babies the women were carrying. It turned out it wasn't: The drug caused miscarriages or severe, usually lethal birth defects. Many thousands of babies died in the womb. Another 10,000 suffered a range of maladies, including shocking deformities.

The hysteria that followed forever changed the public image of the pharmaceutical industry. The drug was never available in the United States (thanks largely to the heroically skeptical FDA doctor Frances Oldham Kelsey), but by 1962 the U.S. public was deeply shaken and demanded safeguards against the possibility that such a dangerous drug could be available here. In a gesture of bipartisan panic, the House and Senate grabbed Kefauver's bill and added it as the Drug Efficacy Amendment to the Federal Food, Drug, and Cosmetic Act. It passed it in one day—possibly the only time this has ever happened in the history of Congress, excepting declarations of war. There would now be three required phases to a drug trial. In Phase I, a treatment is tested on a small group of people to gauge the right dosage of a drug and see how well it works. In Phase II it's given to a larger group to see if it's safe. And in Phase III it's compared with either a placebo or the current standard of care to prove it's effective. (There is also a Phase IV occasionally done once the drug is on the market to look at long-term use.)

Suddenly drugs were required not only to be safe but also to be shown to work better than a placebo. Which turned out to be a tall order. For common conditions like pain and depression, the placebo rate could be north of 80 percent. I've seen smaller studies where that number is essentially 100 percent—*all* the people in the placebo group felt better after taking it, negating the need for the drug at all. It turns out that certain conditions that respond well to placebos come up with shocking regularity: pain, anxiety, depression, irritable bowel syndrome,[4] addiction, nausea, and Parkinson's disease. (As we shall see, there are good reasons why these and not other conditions, like cancer or Alzheimer's disease, allow for seemingly miraculous cures through placebo response.)

But scientists wouldn't understand these things for decades. After Kefauver's bill there was the more immediate problem that no one knew which of the drugs they were already taking were effective. So in 1963 the FDA created the Drug Efficacy Study Implementation, or DESI, a program that retested thousands of drugs to see whether they actually did what they said they did. By 1984 more than *one thousand* drugs were taken off the market, having lost out to placebos. (To date, DESI has not completed its work, meaning it's possible that a drug you're using may be no more effective than a placebo.) The placebo control is one of the main reasons why drugs are so expensive to bring to market.

In many ways, this moment marked the true beginning of modern medicine: For the first time in history there was a law stating that, to be allowed on the market, a drug had to *beat* something. From here

---

4 Irritable bowel syndrome, or IBS, is essentially a catchall term for mysterious painful stomach conditions. No one knows what causes it, but it can vary in severity from annoying to absolutely crippling. Somewhere between a tenth and a quarter of people in the world probably suffer from it, mostly female. If you don't have IBS, there's a good chance you know someone who does.

on, every new pharmaceutical now has to be measured against the effect of a placebo treatment. Such medicine is often referred to as "evidence based," which basically translates as the ability to beat a placebo.

So you would think there would be entire medical school departments devoted to the study of the placebo effect, that Big Pharma would have initiated a massive research effort, that placebo science would be taught in every medical school and chemistry lab. But no. Until recently, not a single institute or concerted effort in the United States was aimed at what essentially is the cornerstone of drugmaking: the placebo effect. The basis of modern medicine was basically ignored. Why? Because placebos are still largely viewed as a nuisance—a bizarre psychological reaction that affects weak and gullible people and keeps the real patients from getting the drugs that they need. But today that view is radically changing.

The only way we have to separate an effective treatment from an ineffective one—and the best metric we have for judging the potency of a drug or procedure—is the randomized, placebo-controlled trial. Yet many drug companies continue to look at placebo responses as a nuisance to be overcome, rather than as an important phenomenon to be understood and exploited. They're squeamish about discussing them. And really, who can blame them? The last thing a drugmaker wants to do is bring attention to the fact that so many of its products—after years of intense research and development—perform no better than a placebo does. If a drug fails, it's best to pretend it never existed. If it succeeds, it's best not to draw attention to how close it came to failing.

But as soon as a drug is approved and hits the market, placebos become the company's best friend. You can see it in the marketing, the commercials, even the look of the pill itself. All are designed to increase your confidence in the product and thus in the ever present placebo effect.

Think about the marketing for a stomach medication. A commercial might show a red, inflamed stomach, then a cool, stabilizing drug coating the walls and making everything OK. Or a headache-medicine ad might show a pill releasing tiny colorful dots that go straight to the throbbing head and relieve the pain. The images are catchy but still vaguely scientific—like a high school biology textbook redesigned by a high-priced ad firm. But that soothing, science-y feel helps bolster your confidence in the drug. When a drug is being developed, expectation and the placebo effect are a hindrance. But when it comes time to sell it, nothing helps it to work as much as our own minds.

• • •

After months of learning about the bizarre history of placebos, I couldn't help wondering what a modern placebo based on vivid storytelling would look like. I wanted to get a glimpse of the kind of charged atmosphere that drove Mesmer's patients into fits or the storytelling that led Hahnemann's patients to find healing in a glass of water. I wanted to see expectation tweaked in real time. So I seek out a master of suggestion.

On the eastern coast of Mexico in the state of Veracruz, just above the Yucatán Peninsula and overlooking a bucolic lake, is a little colonial town called Catemaco. It had very little modern medicine for much of the 20th century (though, ironically, the movie *Medicine Man,* about finding the cure for cancer in a remote Amazon forest, was filmed here). Its people trace their heritage back 2,500 years to the first large civilization in Mesoamerica, called the Olmecs. Many continued to rely on traditional healers long after much of the country had made the shift to Western medicine.

Lineage and tradition are important here, as are the region's famous *brujos,* or witches. (I suppose a more precise translation might be "warlock" since most of them are men.) Brujos have a long tradition throughout Mexico, often blending shamanistic powers of the spirit world, Catholicism, and good old-fashioned health advice. Some are known for their use of hallucinogenic drugs in healing, others for their sweat lodges, others for sacrificing chickens alongside cans of Coke. But none are as renowned as the Catemaco brujos. I'd heard stories of massive pentagram-shaped bonfires and dancing madmen who spit all over you as a blessing. So naturally that's where I went to understand the roots of modern placebo storytelling.

There are, however, no spitting madmen in the waiting room of a modern brujo. The office is in a bright green house in a residential part of town, and looks like an antiseptic cross between a doctor's office and my grandmother's living room. About 10 people sit in chairs reading magazines or watching soccer on the TV. I'm waiting to see Emilio Rosario Organista, second-generation healer and head of the town brujo council. It's not the dark bat-infested lair I had hoped for—it's a tidy little room that smells of hospital disinfectant and has plastic amulets and glass crystals in neat little rows on shelves, like cans of mousse at a salon.

After an hour or so, Rosario invites me back, past the kitchen, to his office. As witch doctors go, he looks more doctor than witch—wearing all white and sporting a neat mustache and short, heavily gelled hair. Half his office is filled by an altar that looks like a Christmas tree exploded, with crucifixes, paintings of saints, and flowers surrounded by hundreds of blinking colored lights. Nailed to the back of his door he has another crucifix, with a jacket hanger dangling from Christ's foot.

I tell him I'm here for a simple *limpia*, a cleaning of my spirit. He grabs an egg, a bunch of basil, and a couple of plastic squirt bottles filled with what he says are envy blockers, bad-energy protection, and a liquid that makes wealth (they smell a little like eucalyptus, rose, and musk). I'm amazed at how orderly and clean everything is. Then he goes to work. He tells me that this is not a Christian ceremony but has me recite the Lord's Prayer anyway, replacing the last line with "to cast out the bad." Though I am fully dressed, he splashes me with water running off the basil, rubs the uncracked egg over me from head to toe, and squirts me liberally with the eucalyptus (which feels a little like taking a bath in BenGay). He stops at my left knee and asks cryptically if it is hurting me. It's not.

After blessing me, he cracks the egg into water and takes a quick look at it. He tut-tuts a bit and points to some bubbles that formed between the water and strands of egg white. He announces that this means there is an envious colleague casting black magic my way. This person is praying for me to get pain, especially in my head and the back of my neck. This person also wants my business to fail. He describes him as a well-muscled white guy who comes to my shoulder. Immediately I think of my photographer friend who's working with me on a project in Baja. Could he secretly be envious of me and wishing me ill? Well, no. For one, he's a photographer and I'm a writer, and our fortunes are linked. Plus, if I had neck problems, he would be out a boxing partner. But I am struck by how quickly my mind finds someone who fits the brujo's vague description. And I remind myself to keep an eye out just in case.

Rosario says that for an extra $25 I can get an amulet that he had blessed for me to put in my pocket to keep me safe from back and knee pain. Furthermore, if I give him a photo of myself, my name, and my birthday, he will pray for me regularly until something good happens to me. When it does—new job, whatever—I can send him whatever amount of money I think is best. I'd be lying if I say I'm not tempted. It's such an obvious scam, yet he acts as if it is the most natural thing ever. As if I've already done it in spirit and all that's necessary is the passing of bills. I decline both offers and give him the 500 pesos (about $35) I have promised.

Then it hits me. I was so busy looking for an exotic theater like Mesmer's or something out of *Harry Potter* that I completely missed the theater Rosario was using. It was the theater of medicine. Modern-day medicine.

Twenty years ago, Mexican journalists tell me, you could still find an "authentic" dancing, spitting witch doctor. But, as I've said, expectation is based on confidence. And the things that inspire confidence change with the culture. What has changed in Catemaco over the last generation? Conventional medicine came to town. Whereas chicken feathers and performance inspired confidence before, brujos today have adapted to the times and have mixed white lab coats and antiseptic spray bottles with powerful Christian and pagan images to tap into their patients' expectations.

Whereas his father might have used shock and fear, Rosario now uses the trappings of hospitals—white clothes, waiting room, and antiseptic smells—to tap into expectation. He is confident, makes eye contact, and smiles warmly while using strange jargon. Most of all, he focuses on pain. Sure, he sprinkles in a little bit of mysticism—the masks, the religious overtones—but the image he wants you to have is of a doctor. A regular medical doctor. It's brilliant.

● ● ●

Placebos and expectation are part of all medicine. They kick in the moment we swallow that pill and the moment we step into the doctor's office and see that white coat. None of us is immune to it, and those who fall under its spell aren't weak or gullible. This is who we are.

After 2,000 years as an eccentric medical mystery, placebo effects are starting to take shape out of the fog. But although these tricks work on everyone, they do not work the same for everyone. Some people look at Rosario and see a caring and capable community healer, while others see a scam artist with a handful of basil. Some see homeopathy as a tested and proven form of personalized medicine. Others see water in a fancy vial.

Everyone's door to expectation has a different key, and everyone is suggestible in a slightly different way. But once that door is unlocked, we have access to an amazing power to heal ourselves. For all human history, this bizarre thing—that Hippocrates warned us about, that Avicenna tried to screen out, that Mesmer capitalized on, that Jellinek dismissed, and that obliterated 1,000 modern medicines—was the brain's own method of self-medication.

Now that we've looked at the keys to the door, let's turn the lock and take a look inside the room beyond. Let's see how this pharmacy inside our own heads works.

CHAPTER TWO

Meet *Your* Inner Pharmacist

Each patient carries his own doctor inside of him.

—Albert Schweitzer, observing a
witch doctor at work

I'M NOT OVERLY FOND OF PAIN. As a kid, I cried when I got bee stings and I have never gone in for masochistic machismo like holding my hand over a candle, getting tattoos, or listening to a Justin Bieber album from start to finish. But I find pain utterly fascinating. Ostensibly, it evolved as a way for your body to tell the brain that something is wrong—your foot is broken, you have been bitten by a snake, a mastodon is stomping on you. But scientists aren't really sure what pain looks like within the brain. Sure, give a good neurologist a brain scan of someone in pain, and he can point out the active regions that clearly show it. "Ah, the anterior cingulate cortex is active. That's due to the pain." But if you give that same specialist (with a few notable exceptions) a scan of a brain without revealing what the person was experiencing at that moment, he probably can't tell you if the person is in pain.

What's more, long after an injury is gone, the pain can hang around, like an uninvited guest sleeping on your couch. Doctors call this chronic pain, and in many ways it's the great overlooked epidemic of our time. According to the Institute of Medicine of the National Academies, 100 million Americans suffer from chronic pain—almost one in three of us. A little less than half of chronic pain sufferers say it disrupts sleep. Most have trouble concentrating, get depressed, and have less energy because of their pain. The medical bills and lost workdays from chronic pain in the United States tally up to $635 billion per year. (By comparison, the entire movie industry directly generates only $9.4 billion in U.S. sales.)

Chronic pain also responds exceptionally well to placebos. In fact, pain might be the signature placebo-prone condition in the world today. This makes it especially easy to relieve with unproven treatments, and it also makes it hard to prove that treatments aren't placebos. Therefore, it's very difficult for drug companies to come up with new drugs to treat the millions of people suffering from pain.

My fascination with placebos and pain brought me to the National Institutes of Health complex. If you were to design an evil, faceless government center for mad scientists, it would look just like the NIH campus in Washington, D.C. It's so sprawling that many employees drive golf carts to get around. The buildings are stark, blocky affairs built of identical red bricks. Several spout ominous fumes.

Despite the Orwellian ambiance, this campus is something of a modern miracle generator. Since the Clinical Center opened in 1953, more than 480,000 people like me have walked through its doors to participate in medical research. Scientists there helped develop chemotherapy, proved that lithium works as a mood stabilizer, and administered the first treatment of AZT for AIDS patients. But I'm not here for any of those fancy experiments with millions of dollars and thousands of subjects. I'm here for pain. Specifically, to understand how it interacts with placebos—and maybe even to feel a little of it.

Luana Colloca's laboratory is tucked into a small corner of the massive and ominous-sounding "Building 10" in the center of the campus. Colloca has warm eyes and a level gaze, with glasses that occasionally slip down her nose and a sort of bashfully nerdy bedside manner punctuated by sudden mischievous smiles. A protégé of the eminent Italian placebo researcher Fabrizio Benedetti, she speaks with a thick Italian accent and has a habit of answering questions by politely saying, "Correct." Perhaps it's that gentle authority that makes me go through with her experiment, which involves me getting electric shocks over and over again.

Her lab is small and tidy. I am relieved and a little disappointed to find that the seat where I will be shocked is just an ordinary office chair, nothing like the fanciful electric chair in *The Green Mile*. She slips out for a second as her assistant tapes sensors and little metal tabs attached to cables to my eyebrow, chest, hands, and left wrist. Then she returns wearing a white lab coat and explains that I'm attached to electrodes that will deliver a shock while sensors measure my reaction—sweating, flinching, heartbeat, and the like. On my left hand are two differently shaped electrodes that will deliver the jolts of electricity.

Colloca points to two devices taped to my left hand. One, on my hand, will deliver the shock. The other, on my middle finger, she says, will tap into A-B fibers in my hand that will occasionally interrupt the shocks, nearly cutting the pain altogether—a kind of electrical crossing guard halting traffic. So the difference between the weak shock and the powerful shock will be that one has the crossing guard, while the other does not. I'll know which one is coming via a screen that will turn green when the A-B fibers are blocking the pain and red when they are not.

Placebo studies often carry some form of deception, and I'm determined to spot it. But the threat of imminent pain is acutely focusing, and as soon as the electrodes are attached, they get all my attention. And as soon as that first shock hits, I forget about everything except my left hand. Getting a small shock feels like a pinprick or a pinch, but a bigger shock doesn't feel like a bigger pinprick. It's more like a dull squeeze wrapped in fire, localized in my hand but seemingly all over my body as well. Colloca slowly increases the strength of the shock, working me up a scale of 1 to 10 (10 being the "worst tolerable pain"), testing my pain threshold. At 6 my foot twitches a little and I can honestly say I am quite perturbed.

"How is that? Seven? Eight?" she asks gently.

"No, I . . . 6? It hurt. I really didn't like it," I reply.

"Are you comfortable to do this several times?"

"Uhhh . . . yeah, sure. I didn't like it," I say, laughing nervously.

She nods and goes into the next room, and we get started. The computer screen in front of me blinks green for number 1 and red for the big number 6. When the A-B nerve fibers are triggered, the shock isn't that bad, but I quickly learn to dread the red screen. It's probably not technically torture, but it *really* hurts. And my foot twitches each time. When the red screen appears, I try to count how many seconds before the jolt—bracing for the hit—but it always catches me by surprise. This goes on for two rounds of 12 shocks each.

On the third round I notice that the green shock has gotten slightly worse—maybe from a 1 to a 2—and I wonder if I have somehow short-circuited the A-B nerve blocker in my hand. We run through 11 more and then the torture session is over. Colloca comes back in, all smiles. She starts by telling me my pain threshold was smack in the middle of the bell curve for pain, 100 hertz of electricity. Interestingly, it seems there are some people who can't take even the slightest touch of electricity and others who have such a high tolerance that you cannot legally shock them enough to even cause pain. I imagine a hulking volunteer in a sheepskin jerkin who feels no pain—and am happy to be in the middle. Then Colloca points to a sheet of paper showing my third round and drops the bomb.

"In Block 3, we used green and red both at 100 hertz. You felt the green as less painful, compared to the red, when actually you received exactly the same," she says and then flashes a mischievous smile. "So that is the placebo effect. It's a pity [you're not in the trial and] we can't use your data because you are a very good placebo responder."

It takes me a second to process. First—what the hell?—she jacked me at full strength for 12 shocks in a row? Is that legal? But every time I saw the green screen, I swear I felt less pain. A *lot* less. I'm not an idiot—I can tell the difference between a pinprick and squeezing fire. Second, my foot didn't twitch when I saw the green screen. It was the electrode on my finger—the one that tapped my A-B fibers and was cutting my pain. Colloca smiles and says there never was any magic pain-lessening wire. She takes the cord leading from my finger and shows me the other end; it's just duct-taped to the back of a machine. It was my own brain, sparked by the green screen, that was cutting down my pain.

I walk out of the lab stunned. I just experienced the magic of the placebo on the human brain.

● ● ●

In real life, placebo responses can be triggered by many things—the desire to please a doctor, for instance, or just to get better. When do you usually go to the doctor? Usually when you are at your worst. And what happens after you are at your worst? You get better. Believe it or not, this "regression to the mean" is its own kind of placebo response. But that day in Colloca's lab was not some conceptual or psychological trick, nor was it regression to the mean. It felt like real pain relief.

It turns out that what happened to me that day was something that has slowly brought placebos from annoying curiosity to a vibrant and crucial area of research. Henry Beecher and Lou Lasagna understood that placebos were important, but they had no idea how they work. Many scientists have noted that people who suffer from pain and certain other afflictions—depression, anxiety, irritable bowels, nausea, and addiction—seem more likely than others to experience placebo effects. This suggests that there has to be some kind of physical process, some neurochemical mechanism, at work. After all, if placebos were caused by the patient just trying to please the doctor, they would be the same across all afflictions. There has to be a mechanism at work in some ailments and not others. What's happening chemically in the brain when placebos are working?

For thousands of years, humans have been taking opium-based painkillers. Indeed, opium might have even been the world's first painkiller. It's the perfect drug: If you are in pain, it takes the pain away; and if you aren't, it makes you as high as a weather balloon. Laudanum, probably the most famous opium tincture, goes back to the 1500s and was popular well into the 1900s. (There were even opium-laced tampons in the 19th century.) Why does it work so well? In the early 1970s, using animal brains, scientists discovered that our brains seem to have special receptors specifically adapted to accept and process opium, which is partly why it's also so addictive. It didn't take these scientists long to then ask the obvious question: Why would we have receptors for a drug that exists only in poppy plants? Unless . . . our brains make something like it as well.

The answer to that question came from a team in Scotland in 1975: Humans do have a form of homemade opioids called endorphins— our own little hidden opium dens tucked away in our brains. Opioids play a number of roles in our brain, such as regulating circadian rhythms, appetite, and body temperature. And they are the primary chemicals that make sex feel so good. Inspired by this discovery of brain-generated opium-like chemicals, two San Francisco neurologists, Jon Levine and Howard Fields, conducted a simple experiment with people in pain after dental surgery. They wanted to see if these newfangled endorphins might be involved in the placebo effect.

The plan was to give a group of patients who had recently had a dental procedure either a placebo or naloxone, a drug that blocks the brain's opioids, and tell all of them they were receiving a painkiller. Essentially, one group was getting nothing and the other less than nothing. As expected, many of those who got the placebo felt less pain, just as I felt less pain whenever I saw a green screen in Colloca's lab. Meanwhile, the naloxone group was still miserable, as their own natural opioid generator was being blocked. Then, when naloxone was given to the placebo group, they joined the other half in feeling miserable again. Essentially, they had made the placebo effect evaporate with a drug. The study elegantly showed that pain placebos work because the brain self-medicates with opioid drugs.

Today, Levine and Fields's work is seen as a landmark study that defines the modern placebo. But at the time, few scientists grasped the implications. Throughout the 1980s and part of the '90s, placebo research continued as a kind of fringe field that appealed to a few iconoclastic academics. One of the biggest was Irving Kirsch, a former professional violinist and Vietnam War activist who took up psychology out of a philosophical curiosity about the brain. Over the past three decades, his work has helped crystallize the role of opioids' brain pathways in placebo responses.

Kirsch mentored Ted Kaptchuk, a researcher who earned a Chinese doctorate in Eastern medicine and was an expert in acupuncture and other alternative therapies; he transferred this into an enduring interest in how the brain affects the body. The two set up a research lab at Harvard, and for a long time their names have been pretty much synonymous with placebo research. Kaptchuk's work spans many complicated aspects of placebo research—genetic, biochemical—but my favorite study of his is a relatively simple one. He handed patients a pill and told them it was a placebo. He added that placebos have been shown to be very effective against all manner of conditions, et cetera, et cetera. And when they took the pill, it still worked! Not as well as a secret placebo—but it worked, even though the people taking it knew it wasn't real.

The reason why a placebo works has nothing to do with psychology or opinions or weakness, but rather a chemical interaction outside our control in the brain. This is not philosophy; this is brain science. But studying the brain is not like studying any other organ in the body. It's far more complicated. Scientists can only study it in several limited, incomplete ways.

Let me offer a metaphor for the brain to help you understand the challenges brain scientists face. Imagine your brain is one giant football stadium, with each person being a brain cell, or a neuron. Now imagine a group of aliens who know nothing about human language or culture trying to understand the rules of the game just by watching the crowds in the stadium.

How should they start? How about with what the people are wearing? Clearly blue is important to one tribe, while orange is key for the other. How about behavior? Some people will be rooting for one team, the rest for the other. Lots of blue fans will be loud all at once, but it won't keep the orange ones quiet or keep their cheerleaders from dancing. Some in the stadium won't be rooting for anyone, only trying to impress their dates or clients. Others will be focused on selling hot dogs, stamping tickets, or pouring beer. Then there is the press box, business office, and locker room, where people seem totally unconnected with what's happening on the field.

What is the best thing to measure? Noise level? How much money people spend or make? How many trips they take to the bathroom? Then what? Should the aliens pick a few individual fans and study them really carefully? Or break the stadium into parts and try to gather general ideas? Perhaps people in the box seats act differently from those in the bleachers. Perhaps the section between LL and MM on the upper deck just above the 25-yard line is particularly important.

It's a big mess. But instead of holding 67,000 people, imagine a stadium that hosts more than 85 billion. That's about 1.2 million U.S. football stadiums. And instead of just one game, imagine multiple events are going on at the same time. Say, a rock concert, a political rally, and, I don't know, maybe a comic book convention. And most fans seem to be watching more than one event at once.

That's your brain, in a nutshell.

The scientist's job is to wade through all that confusion and try to discover something useful. No matter what he chooses to focus on—the movement of blood, electrical pulses, glucose uptake—there will always be a boggling amount of extra noise. Given that complexity, the chance of seeing something as subtle as a placebo response is pretty thin.

In 2002, scientists from Sweden's prestigious Karolinska Institute demonstrated that a person in pain can release his own opioids to ease that pain. Two years later, psychology Ph.D. student Tor Wager took this this study one step further in an amazing study that began as just a side interest to his Ph.D. research.

"When I started grad school, there was this idea that there were certain areas that people *should* study," he says. Placebos were not in that group. Sure, it was fine for famous scientists or the Dalai Lama to wax poetic about mind-body interactions, but not for a young scientist deciding on a career path. Colleagues warned Wager that the field was "flaky" and "not kosher."

But Wager had a deep, personal connection to the topic. Like me, he was raised in Christian Science and had seen these things work up close, as I had. In fact, when I first saw his name on the list of attendees at a 2009 brain conference, it stopped me in my tracks. You see, Wager and I had attended the same tiny college in Elsah, Illinois—a college exclusively for Christian Scientists. What, I wondered, was a Christian Scientist doing delivering the keynote at a brain meeting?

Wager studying placebos is a little like a former Catholic studying the brain's response to guilt. And although he has since fallen away from Christian Science, the same way I have, that same nagging fascination with mental healing had stuck with him, as it had with me. He had seen friends and family members rely completely on the power of the mind for their health and had heard miraculous-sounding tales of instantaneous recovery. He wasn't willing to chalk all that up to some kind of gullible self-delusion.

"It's kind of hard to reconcile [religion with] believing in things based on evidence, because they're fundamentally different," Wager said during our first conversation. He's a shy, self-effacing guy with a powerful frame, close-cut brown hair, and sleepy eyes. "I always felt that Christian Scientists should be physicians. [Founder] Mary Baker Eddy used morphine. I don't think Christian Science started out as this 'you're either with us or against us' kind of thing."

Wager became an early adopter of the growing field of brain imaging, especially functional magnetic resonance imaging, or fMRI, which measures blood moving to activate parts of the brain as they engage. Now, fMRI doesn't actually measure activity, just blood flow. And not really even that—just blood oxygen levels. In the stadium analogy, think of it as beer (or blood alcohol levels, if you prefer). The amount of beer that various sections are drinking predicts what ones will be making the most noise. So if you can't measure noise, you measure the movement of beer. But remember, the brain is really big.

Scientists measure brain activity in voxels, which are kind of like pixels on a computer screen that combine to make a picture. But a single voxel has some 630,000 neurons in it (and four times as many cells connecting them to each other). In other words, the smallest unit scientists can use to measure an indirect form of brain activity contains about 9.4 football stadiums.

Add to that all the other noise, which makes it *really* hard to say what's actually going on in a brain scanned by an fMRI machine. Over the past decade and a half, scientists and the media have gone a little nuts with fMRI, claiming to have found parts of the brain responsible for things like political affiliation. Often these studies turn out to be little more than fancy guesswork. After all, there are more neurons in the brain than stars in our galaxy.[5] Understanding signals in such a complex organ, statistically speaking, is like trying to track every human on Earth.

Wager was aware of fMRI's limitations early on, and so became a student of the arcane world of the statistics involved in separating useful fMRI data from background noise. Then he set up two simple experiments to try to capture the placebo effect in action. First was the electric shock experiment. Subjects saw either a red or a blue spiral on a screen warning them they would get either a strong or a mild shock, which would hit between 3 and 12 seconds later to keep them off guard (and build expectation). Once they understood the ground rules, Wager gave them two creams, explaining that one was designed to reduce the pain and the other was a placebo, and they ran the test again. In fact, both were placebos. Yet amazingly, people said they felt less pain with the "active" cream!

The second experiment used a burning heat pad that seared the skin for a brutal 20 seconds. This time, the screen just read, "Get

---

5 Fun fact: This statistic is bandied about online a lot, and people often mistakenly say "universe" instead of "galaxy." If your brain had as many neurons as stars in the universe, it would weigh about 1.5 billion tons.

Ready!" and then the pad heated up. As in the other trial, the subjects put placebo and pain-killing creams, both of which were actually placebos, on their arms. But this time Wager surreptitiously lowered the temperature of the heat pad on the fake "active" cream, fooling the subjects into thinking that the cream was reducing the level of pain they felt. Then, in the last phase (as Colloca had with my shocks), he kept the temperature high.

As in any placebo study, researchers kept careful records of how much pain the subjects reported feeling. Normally, when the subjects reported feeling less pain with placebo creams, it would have been easy to shrug and say that people are easy to deceive and will say whatever they think the scientist wants to hear. But Wager also had their fMRI brain scans. Something surprising happened when he analyzed the data: What people said about their pain tracked perfectly with the activation of several parts of the brain associated with pain, such as the anterior cingulate cortex (which plays a role in emotions, reward systems, and empathy), the thalamus (which handles sensory perception and alertness), and the insula (which is related to consciousness and perception). Those reporting less pain from the placebo effect showed less activity in key pain-related brain regions. And those who felt less of the placebo showed more. People were not imagining less pain; they were feeling it.

Wager's study not only conclusively showed that the placebo effect is a real phenomenon in the brain; it also showed that people experiencing a placebo effect aren't crazy or deluded or gullible. Most important, Wager observed the route that the placebo response takes from anticipation to the release of drugs. Normally, pain signals begin in the more primitive base of the brain (relaying information from wherever in the body the pain starts) and radiate outward. What he saw was backward, with the pain signals starting in the prefrontal cortex—the most advanced logic center of the brain—and working back to the more primitive regions. This seemed to suggest a sort of collision of information: half originating in the body as pain, and half originating in the advanced part of the brain as expectation. And whatever comes out of that collision is what you feel.

What had begun as a side project quickly became an obsession. Wager submitted his placebo findings to the prestigious journal *Science*. Then he interviewed for an assistant professorship at Columbia University. When asked what he was planning to study, rather than his actual research area of visual perception, Wager took a deep breath and said, "Placebos." In some circles this was akin to telling a biology department you planned to study Sasquatch. But the Columbia professors decided to give the kid a chance.

Not long after, *Science* made the same call and published his paper in 2004. With that and the Karolinska Institute study, placebos were officially out of the closet. Today, Wager's *Science* paper has been referenced in hundreds of other prestigious research journals and is often credited with anointing placebos as a true neurochemical phenomenon, not mere self-delusion.

Together these scientists—from Beecher to Kirsch to Benedetti to Wager to Colloca—have managed to cobble together a picture of what placebos look like in the brain. Pain, like any sensation, starts in the body, goes up the spine, and then travels to the deeper brain structures that distribute that information to places like the prefrontal cortex, where we can contemplate it. Placebos, on the other hand, seem to start in the prefrontal cortex (just behind your right temple) and go *backward*. They work their way to parts of the brain that handle opioid production and release chemicals that dull the pain. They also seem to tamp down activity in the parts of the brain that recognize pain in the first place. And you feel better. All in a fraction of a second.

● ● ●

So what does this mean for you and me? Inside us is an expectation-fueled suite of drugs posed to change how we see painful experiences. But can we harness those drugs? It turns out we already do. Every time you center your chakras or get a blessing from the local shaman, you are engaging your expectation pharmacy. But even among alternative medicines, not all are created equal.

Enter my very favorite placebo treatment, acupuncture. As with so many forms of folk medicine, acupuncture doesn't reliably outperform a placebo. When it does, it's for especially placebo-prone conditions like pain or nausea. But although acupuncture doesn't often outperform placebos, it still performs really well, and many respected scientists are not yet ready to label it strictly brain chemistry. Ted Kaptchuk even found that the brain's response to acupuncture is markedly different than it is to other placebos. It performs so well, it seems to be in its own class of placebo.

Naturally I had to try it.

When I show up to an acupuncture studio a few miles from my house, I feel a little nervous. My acupuncturist is a beefy, clean-cut American from the Bay Area who graduated from a well-respected Chinese medicine school and has been practicing for about two years. I identify myself as a journalist and tell him I'm there to treat a chronic pain condition in my forearm caused by rock climbing and typing with bad posture. He proceeds to ask me a barrage of questions about my overall mental, physical, and sexual health that have nothing to do with my forearm.

Of course, I understand that acupuncture involves the sticking of tiny sharp things into your skin, but somehow I still feel surprised when he reaches for individually wrapped pins and starts sticking them in me. Even more surprising, they often hurt going in. About every third or fourth needle feels like it's hitting some kind of knot or nerve in my arm.

He explains that this feeling is related to blockages of either my blood or my chi, the Chinese concept of spiritual energy. When an acupuncturist inserts a needle, he or she is trying to loosen up the blockages, like some kind of spiritual Roto-Rooter. These should not be confused with the electrical energy involved in the nervous system, since nerve fibers are far too small to target with needles this big. And yet, something is clearly happening with my nervous system: Occasionally I feel a tingling sensation moving up my arm, and my finger twitches. And once the needles go in, moving my arm is agony.

After he's done, the acupuncturist walks out of the room while the needles do their work. It's pleasant and relaxing in the room, and I find myself drowsily floating between sleep and consciousness. I am acutely aware of the dull throbbing in my arm. I try to imagine the needles releasing my blockages like dynamite detonating tiny dams in my arm. Lying there listening to recorded nature sounds lulls me into a trance, and one possible mechanism for how acupuncture works occurs to me.

In certain scientific studies (often involving drugs with powerful side effects), the moment subjects realize they aren't having any side effects, they know they are in the placebo group and the effect withers (but still doesn't disappear). So to boost the placebo effect, scientists occasionally give an "active" placebo—a pill that is mostly inert except for some tiny effect, like tingling fingers. The subject feels her fingers tingling and thinks, "Wow, I don't know what it's doing, but it's doing something." Her expectation now reinforced, she's free to have the full placebo response.

Naturally, active placebos are not popular with FDA drug trials because they are expensive, hard to make, and often increase the placebo effect beyond the reach of many prospective drugs. Imagine for a moment that you set up an experiment comparing a painkiller without side effects with an active placebo. Everyone on the placebo would assume they had the drug; those with the drug would assume they had the placebo.

What if acupuncture is an active placebo? What if that tingling sensation in my nerves and pain in my muscles is a message to my brain that this exercise with needles is doing something. That would explain why it performs so well in trials, yet not well enough to reliably beat placebos.

Is my acupuncturist using an active placebo? On one hand, he hasn't seemed too interested in the theater of medicine. He hasn't spun elaborate tales of ancient Chinese mysticism the way I expected him to. He simply asked me a list of questions and started sticking needles in me. But when I asked about which conditions are best suited to acupuncture, he offered up a familiar list: musculoskeletal pain, digestive problems, stress, and sleep issues. There is no question that the acupuncture wheelhouse is pretty well aligned with the placebo wheelhouse.

In the end, it doesn't matter much, since it doesn't work for me. After six weeks of regular acupuncture sessions, I see no improvement in my poor forearm, so I stop going.

● ● ●

How powerful are placebo effects? Well, in some people, they barely register. In others, the opioid dumps can be so powerful that, in essence, they become physically addicted to their own internal opioids, similar in theory to how people once became addicted to laudanum. One provocative theory even suggests that chronic pain might be the result of a brain addicted to its inner pharmacy and, in a sense, looking for a fix.

And it's not just opioids. Over the past few decades, other brain chemicals have been shown to trigger the placebo effect. Your inner pharmacy also stocks endocannabinoids—the same class of chemicals found in marijuana that play a role in pain suppression—and serotonin, which is important in intestinal movements and the primary neurotransmitter involved in feelings of happiness and well-being.

By now you should be noticing a pattern in the drugs that seem most connected with the placebo effect: opioids, cannabinoids, serotonin. These are all needed for the treatment of pain, depression, anxiety, irritable bowels, nausea, and addiction—the conditions that are unusually responsive to placebos.

But there is one more to add to the pile, and it's perhaps the most important chemical in your inner pharmacy: dopamine. If you've heard of dopamine, chances are you know it as a neurotransmitter involved in reward processing. If a colleague walks by your desk and offers you a beautiful slice of cake, you will release a dopamine shot to the nucleus accumbens of your brain. Get some money? Another shot. How about sex? Another, probably larger, shot. But dopamine is far more than an occasional bit of reward bliss. It's also a key player in movement, insulin release, and blood flow. Lack of it may play a role in both schizophrenia and attention deficit disorder. It has the power to intensify nausea, initiate key parts of the immune system, increase urine, and slow down the gastrointestinal tract. It plays a crucial role in attention, memory, cognition, pituitary function (which, in turn, influences hundreds of processes, including lactation, orgasm, and sleep), nausea, and, of course, pain processing.

In short, dopamine is not a neurotransmitter to mess with. The chemistry of the brain is incredibly complicated, but it's not hard to see that dopamine is one of the prime ingredients. It's the brain's puppet master and its board of directors. Dopamine's got friends in almost every part of your body, and if you try to pick a fight with it, well, it can make things uncomfortable for you. But it can also grease the wheels that need greasing. Dopamine, it turns out, is also a huge player in the placebo effect. After all, what's reward without expectation?

When it comes to its effect on such ailments as chronic pain, depression, and sexual dysfunction, it's difficult to untangle dopamine from the other chemicals it interacts with. But there is one that lends itself perfectly to research. Parkinson's disease is a somewhat mysterious and incurable condition whereby neurons deep in the brain responsible for generating dopamine die. Why they die isn't clear, but since dopamine is so important for movement, patients are increasingly unable to walk, stand, or hold a pen without shaking. Their mood devolves into depression and anxiety. They often abuse drugs, gamble compulsively (possibly as a form of self-medication, since their brains are producing less dopamine, which regulates rewards), and if it gets bad enough, develop dementia. Although Parkinson's itself isn't lethal, its sufferers tend to have shortened lives.

Many placebo studies have looked at Parkinson's patients, and what they tend to see is nothing short of amazing. Jon Stoessl at the University of British Columbia in Canada has done the most work by far in this area. In a 2010 study, he and his co-author invited a Parkinson's patient to try a cutting-edge medication and then get their brains scanned using positron emission tomography, or PET, which focuses on the release of chemicals in the brain (as opposed to the fMRI's focus on blood flow). The man came in on a wheelchair. After taking the drug and sitting for the scan, he practically sprinted up the stairs to the debrief room . . . where they informed him that the new drug was a placebo.

The study showed a massive release of dopamine in the brains of people who have very little of it available. It's common for Parkinson's patients to show placebo response north of 50 percent. Interestingly, in this study the dopamine release was highest in people who had been told there was a small chance they might *not* have gotten the drug. It seems that part of placebo's power might come from a sense of hope, as if the gamble of it all heightens the power of a placebo response.

In cases like the man in the wheelchair, the placebo effect is often temporary. It wears off when the brain stops pumping out excess dopamine. But Stoessl wonders if there might not be a permanent version. It's a refrain that occurs again and again in placebo work. Sure, making a momentary electric shock disappear is cool, but what does that mean for chronic pain sufferers? Can you erase years of agony, as Colloca erased the shock to my hand? After all, a placebo tinkers with the fundamental purpose of your brain—its prediction function. If it can lead that function astray temporarily, might it lead it astray permanently?

● ● ●

Hoping to realize that possibility, pain experts stymied by seemingly unbeatable pain conditions have been turning to placebo researchers over the past few years. One of those people is Sean Mackey, a Stanford University pain researcher who is one of the field's fastest rising stars.

"We are moving away from 'this is all just psychological BS' to 'there is really something to it,' " he says, sitting in a small plaza outside Stanford's Pain Management Center. "Psychology is neuroscience."

Mackey has studied the relationship between feeling pain and watching others feel pain. He has also found tentative similarities between taking painkillers and being in love, as well as between physical pain and an upsetting romantic breakup. He pioneered a therapy that allowed pain patients to see their own brain activity in real time through an fMRI machine as they attempted to change their perception of their pain. He says all this work is driven to some extent by his own failure.

"The sad fact is that I am right about 40 percent of the time. Maybe on a good day 50 percent. If you're playing baseball, you're making millions. If you're a physician, it's not a lot to brag about," he says.

"I'm pretty good at what I do, but the fact is that it's a lot of trial and error that we do with patients. It frustrates them; it frustrates us."

Mackey says scientists don't really know what pain is, let alone why one person ends up with horrible pain after a surgery and someone else doesn't. In the beginning of his career he focused on radial nerves and nerve endings—basically, the part of the nervous system that actually detects the pain in your hand or your knee. But over time, he realized that a lot of pain isn't about the nerve endings but about how the impulses are received and processed by the brain. Especially when those impulses refuse to stop. He says that initially, pain is a warning system, but if it becomes chronic, it turns into something else: a sort of continual feedback loop.

"Many people eventually stop coding the danger signal. But some people don't seem to," he says. "It's a problem of accepting, coding, interpreting, and responding."

In other words, prediction. Expectation. No one told the brain that it's no longer in danger, so it keeps expecting danger and warning the body. This is why anxiety, depression, and stress are so closely linked to chronic pain. The game becomes finding ways to tell the brain it's OK to relax, even if that means tricking it. Mackey and other pain doctors can do this using pain blockers that stop the warning messages from transmitting, thus forcing the brain to realize it's no longer in pain.[6]

So is there a way to enhance the placebo effect, even make it permanent? This seems to be the biggest question in placebo research today. Karin Jensen, a placebo researcher at Harvard, thinks the answer might lie in the subconscious. Remember that most researchers rely

---

6 There was another experiment along these lines at the University of California, San Diego, whereby amputees suffering from phantom-limb pain used mirrors carefully positioned to make it look as if the arm or leg were still in place. Soon the brain realizes there is no more danger, and the pain stops.

on some form of conditioning to elicit a response like the one I experienced at NIH. What if that conditioning could program us to self-medicate without our knowing?

Jensen is in her mid-30s and has bright blond hair and large blue eyes. First in her native Sweden and now in Boston, she has built a career out of coming up with creative ways to fool the brain. In 2015 she published an experiment that showed how your brain can self-medicate even when you are not paying attention. She set up a two-pronged experiment in which subjects wore a painful heat pad that flared up whenever they saw a picture of a certain face (let's call him Bob) and died down when they saw another, similar face (we'll call him Bill). The brain quickly learns that Bob is bad and Bill is good.

Then Jensen took things up a notch. Once the relationship was ingrained in the subject, she turned the heat to somewhere in the middle. This time, she showed the picture for only a fraction of a second, so subjects could barely identify the face. The subconscious mind could spot the difference, but the conscious mind could not. Yet people continued to feel more pain with Bob and less with Bill, even when they couldn't tell one from the other. When Jensen brought me to her Harvard lab and showed me what the subjects had seen, I quickly saw that it's impossible to separate one image from the next—partly because the images went by too quickly, and partly because Bob and Bill looked similar enough to be brothers. But our brains are good at recognizing faces, and the experiment showed that some part of my brain was capturing those images—and, though I was not aware of it, linking each with the conditioned pain experience. With enough practice, subjects can unconsciously trigger the placebo effect with the flash of one face, even though their conscious mind has no idea it's happening. (It's a little like Ted Kaptchuk's experiment, in which he told people they were getting placebos.

Consciously they knew nothing was in the pill, but unconsciously their inner pharmacy was still dispensing drugs.)

When it comes to boosting placebos, we have active placebos and the subtle observations of the subconscious. But there might be another, time-tested way to do it. In the summer of 2015 I visit Tor Wager's lab at the foot of the Rocky Mountains. After his remarkable entrée into science, I expect him to be firmly planted in the Ivy League, battling it out for top grants and journals. But he prefers the slower pace and the stunning natural setting of the University of Colorado. Like so many people who study placebos, he's an easy guy to like.

The work at Wager's lab is split between placebo research and brain imaging around pain. While I'm there, I meet Leonie Koban, one of Wager's students, who has stumbled on another potential game-changer in the world of mind-body healing. Koban started out with a simple idea: How much is the placebo effect altered by peer pressure? Will another person's experience affect yours? She set up an experiment in which people rated various levels of heat pain applied to their arms by a metal pad. After gauging each person's pain threshold, she asked them to rate how much pain they expected to feel before she applied it, but with one crucial added element. They would also be able to see how other people had rated that same pain.

The data mapping other people's reactions was composed of just a few hash marks on the screen. But in essence those marks were saying, "Look, you might think this hurts, but most of the other people who've sat here didn't think it was that big a deal." Or perhaps the reverse: "Everyone else who has done this practically screamed in agony. But don't worry. I'm sure you'll be fine."

As you might expect, those previous reports of pain were totally made up. Yet people who felt a strong pain rated it lower if that's what they thought others had done. And people who were told others had felt a lot of pain rated the pain highly even if it was mild. This peer pressure placebo effect was not only measurable, it was *twice as strong* as the normal placebo effect! Just to be sure no one was fibbing, Koban recorded their skin conductance, which is a physiological response to pain. Whether their pain was real or fake, it was impossible to differentiate from a genuine experience. "It's one of the strongest effects I've ever seen in psychology," Koban told me. "I was surprised. And so was Tor. Because in the beginning he didn't think this would work."

And here's the kicker. There was no need for any kind of Pavlov-style conditioning. People, it seems, are programmed with a preexisting need to go with the herd. In an instant, people tapped into a more powerful placebo response than if they had spent hours conditioning themselves. Let that sink in for a second. Someone else's opinion is not only powerful, it can be more powerful than your own. It can be more powerful than your experience and even more powerful than repeated conditioning. We are hardwired to follow other people's opinions.

There may be some biochemistry to back up this notion. In 2015, Luana Colloca of NIH did an experiment much like the one I participated in but with a crucial difference. I was given a full electric shock but tricked by a green screen into feeling less pain, whereas subjects in this study of Colloca's received a dose of something called vasopressin before they were tricked by a green screen. With this addition, the women in her group experienced a massive placebo response and felt less pain. But vasopressin isn't just a drug; it's also a hormone produced in our bodies. Like its cousin oxytocin, it plays a major role in social interactions between people. In particular, it seems to regulate social communication and conciliatory behavior.

In other words, the same chemicals that draw us together as humans and allow us to live and work together can also boost the placebo response. Imagine if there was a way to harness that power. Imagine if there was a way to amplify it, focus it, and monetize it. By now I shouldn't have to tell you that there already is.

● ● ●

When Mao Zedong came to power in China during the middle of the 20th century, he set about abolishing the imperial-style traditional culture of ancient China. Names were changed, historic sites destroyed, histories pasted over—and most important, religious institutions erased. The one thing he didn't eradicate was the enormously popular—and cost-effective—traditional Chinese medicine, or TCM. Although, according to his personal physician, Mao himself refused TCM and used Western medicine, he allowed the practice to continue, regulated under a separate government agency and standardized across the country.

Thus began a bizarre dual health care system that continues in China to this day. On one side is Western medicine with its MRIs, morphine, surgeries, and so on. On the other is TCM, which treats patients with acupuncture, herbs, animal parts, and massage. Just like conventional medicine, TCM has its own hospitals and drugstores; its students go through extensive schooling (though it's usually not as long as that of their Western-medicine counterparts). Unlike conventional medicine, TCM doesn't run placebo-controlled trials or comparisons against other remedies to see how they work (though outside scientists often do). And no treatment, no matter how arcane or potentially dangerous, has ever been dropped from its repertoire. Every remedy that has ever been used in TCM—from ginseng to rhinoceros horn to mercury—is theoretically just as valid today as it ever was. In other words, evidence is not the primary driver.

As a Westerner, it can be hard to imagine medicine that is not based on scientific evidence, and many outsiders say it's just a clever collection of placebos. There is strong evidence backing this claim. Few, if any, TCM ingredients outperform placebos when tested in the lab, though practitioners counter that the sum of a treatment cannot be measured by its parts. Furthermore, the offerings on display at the pharmacies in China reflect a certain trend: Almost all of them focus on pain, anxiety, lack of energy, or upset stomachs, which we recognize as highly placebo-prone conditions. Yet TCM is still widely popular—not just in China but also around the world. Reports suggest that 75 percent of the Chinese population uses it; it's a point of national pride and one of the country's biggest exports. If the most populous country on Earth has been duped by placebos, they must be pretty good ones.

So I fly to Beijing to meet with Zhang Lin, a practitioner and a teacher at China's biggest and most prestigious TCM university, Capital University of Medicine Sciences.

"In Chinese medicine we don't have 'bacteria.' We don't have this word. We don't have 'virus.' We consider maybe this is the chi or the blood movement," she says. "For Chinese medicine, what we adjust is chi, blood, the yin and the yang."

Modern science cannot measure yin or yang, the Chinese complementary feminine and masculine principles, and no serious scientists—East or West—have been able to demonstrate the existence of chi. Furthermore, Zhang explains that "blood" in the TCM context is more metaphorical than the actual cells and fluid that medical science recognizes. A person's chi, their vital energy, can change with the seasons, the time of day, and a hundred other things. When I ask her how she can prove this, she points to tradition. Over thousands of years TCM has been honed by millions of physicians, evolving naturally over time to where it is today. As with homeopathy, TCM has a coherent story to tell that works perfectly within its own logic but contradicts biology and physics. And as with homeopathic remedies, TCM treatments are often as much about the description of the pain as the physiology.

Zhang tells me about one of her patients, a man from Inner Mongolia who came in with significant digestive problems after months of trying ineffective Western medicines. He was uncomfortable and unable to meet her eyes. After a series of conversations, Zhang realized the problem was not digestion but depression. The two are connected, she says, and the observation actually makes some sense, I suppose: Serotonin and dopamine both play important roles in mood and digestion (though such drugs are not a part of TCM). Zhang prescribed a cocktail of herbs and other ingredients to treat the depression, and the man's stomach issues slowly got better. Each week she'd talk to the man, bring him out of his shell, and tweak his prescription—and each week, he got better. Is it possible the man's belief in TCM—strengthened by a shared belief with millions of other TCM patients—helped cure him? Zhang insists that the efficacy of her work has nothing to do with belief or faith that the treatment will work, but with the treatment itself.

Sitting in Zhang's lovely office in the heart of the world's largest state-sponsored institution of alternative medicine, I think of vasopressin, the drug Colloca has used to boost placebo effects, and Leonie Koban's work with peer pressure. Any time a group of people get together, there's a good chance that vasopressin is flowing. Could it be that the same brain chemistry involved in how we interact with each other actually boosts the placebo effect? Koban found that peer pressure jacks up the placebo effect. Is it such a leap to think that the number of people using a given therapy is not just an effect of how well that therapy works but the *cause* of how well it works? Viewed this way, vasopressin might be the difference between saying, "Take this; it works" and "Take this; a billion people say it works."

If social norms indeed play a role in chemically boosting expectation, then traditional Chinese medicine would be the most powerful placebo the world has ever seen. Imagine the vasopressin release of everyone coming into this hospital, seeing their peers doing the same thing, and knowing that this kind of medicine has helped millions of people for more than 2,000 years. And would this effect be any different for you in a Western hospital?

Zhang tells me a story about a man who wanted to find the best healer in China. He went to the four best that he knew of. Each gave the man a different prescription for the same problem, leading him to assume they were all frauds. But to his surprise, the first remedy actually worked. A year later, the problem (she didn't specify what it was) returned, and out of curiosity, the man tried the second remedy. It worked as well.

For Zhang, the point of the story is that the chemicals in, say, ginseng or deer antler are not as important as the intangible, ineffable quality of the healer. There are many roads, she says, but the destination is the same.

I have to agree—but is it so crazy to think those roads might have a chemical pattern as well? The only thing that remained the same in her tale was the patient. The solution must have come not from the treatments but from his own brain. When I mention this to Zhang, she thinks about it a moment and then says, "Chinese medicine—the theory, the philosophy—is just like the Bible or the Buddha's book. Think of it from this point of view. It's like an artist with three different paintings. Which one is better? Which one is best?"

Zhang says that Western medicine is a straight line—always refining itself, always moving forward—while Chinese medicine is a circle around a fixed dot. The fundamentals never change, just your interpretations of them. Sitting there drinking my third pot of tea, all this starts to sound very familiar. I am reminded for a moment of my parents and their community of faith healers in California. "What you are describing is religion," I say, forgetting for a moment that I'm still in communist China.

She pauses and then, perhaps forgetting herself for a moment too, says, "Um, yes."

Of course, a few herbs in Chinese medicine have yielded valuable drugs—most notably artemisinin, an herb that is effective against malaria and led to a Nobel Prize in medicine. But most efforts to extract useful medications from herbs have been disappointing. So, how have techniques with few demonstrable mechanisms and little efficacy beyond a placebo worked for so many people for so long?

After several days with Zhang, I feel the need to step away from academic discussions and experience TCM firsthand. So I make an appointment at Wang Kai Lang's massage parlor. Located in the old town of Beijing, his office is clean and tidy with white walls, cutaway illustrations of the human body, and a white doctor's coat hanging from a hook. Wang, a charming ball of energy with frizzy, unkempt hair and short, erratic movements, talks in a series of unfinished sentences, one piled onto the next.

We begin with a foot soak in really hot water sprinkled with herbs, while he massages my back and forearms. Then he moves to my feet, where he sets up camp for way, way too long. Using a number of angry little plastic dowels, he pushes, prods, and rubs every tiny muscle in my foot. I'm a huge fan of foot rubs, but this is downright painful. I yelp, grunt, bark, and—I'm ashamed to admit—even squeak once or twice. At one point in Chinese history, loyalty to the party was judged by how well you could hold out under torture. Wang politely makes it clear that I could never be a trusted party member.

According to the theory of Chinese medicine, you can tell a lot about your health by looking at your foot. Each muscle is tied to an organ in the body through meridians, or energy highways. Because the feet and toes are farthest from the heart, they are seen as good diagnostic tools—the 10 little piggies in the coal mine, if you will.

As he works, I tell Wang about the pain in my forearm. He nods and makes guesses about other health problems I might have.

"How is your urinary tract? He wants to know if you have troubles there," my translator says.

"No, my urinary tract is fine. *Agh!*"

"Is your urine yellow?"

"No, it's—*gah, son of a bitch!*—clear and copious," I say, remembering a phrase that describes healthy urine.

"Do you get enough exercise?"

"Yes! *Ungggggggneesh!* I work out regularly. I worked out yesterday."

"He says you need to drink more water. He's very concerned about your urinary tract."

There is no physiological mechanism by which the foot could tell you something about the urinary tract. But that doesn't bother Wang. He's happy in his practice and knows he's helping people (though my arm pain is no better after seeing him). When I ask him how he can be so sure that his work is effective, he has a simple, familiar response: "For so many thousands of years the Chinese people have been the most populous on the Earth, and they have all gone to Chinese medicine to cure their illnesses. How can we doubt it?"

Perhaps that's the answer I've been looking for: *so many people.* If you wanted to boost the serotonin of your depression drug, for example, the best thing you could do would be to seek out other people for whom it had worked.

I think of Leonie Koban's research on peer pressure. "A really good way to increase placebo effects or increase the power of a real medical treatment is to tell people, 'This works for 99 out of 100' or 'This works for millions of people,' " she'd told me. In her experiment, a couple of hash marks on a screen representing people you will never meet are enough to boost the power of the placebo effect beyond even what conditioning can do. Now imagine those hash marks are not mere data but your family, friends, and everyone around you. For thousands of years. And this isn't some vague expectation about a heat pad being slightly more painful than it was a second ago. It's everything you've ever known. How big will the placebo response be then? Enough to sustain an entire shadow medical establishment? Enough to catch on with people all over the world who didn't grow up in this culture, but find confidence in a tradition so old and so popular that its power seems undeniable?

Enough to make the healing permanent?

It certainly seems plausible. It could be that the mere knowledge of millions of people trusting a form of medicine is enough to boost the power of that medicine. It's fair to say that Koban and Colloca have only scratched the surface of how expectation interacts with community. Confidence has power, none more so than the confidence of being in a group. And the more we dig, the more we will see that—just as with opioids and placebos—there are powerful, important chemicals behind that confidence. Vasopressin is not the whole story, but it's a pretty good beginning.

Certainly this feels right to me. It's hard to explain the effect of community and healing to someone who's never experienced it. I remember the power of my Christian Science community in Northern California. Whenever I was sick, our friends and neighbors supported my parents, read stories of other people's healings thousands of miles away, and searched daily for a deeper connection to their faith. It was a powerful narrative of expectation boosted by a tight-knit community of loving people all around me. And it worked.

Outsiders often wonder how people can stay connected to a faith like this—thinking, "Eventually, won't they naturally drift toward solutions that are reinforced by success?" But Christian Science, like

TCM, *is* being reinforced. Humans aren't stupid. Like everyone, Christian Scientists are trying to put their faith in treatments that work.

The results can be stunning. I've seen Christian Science heal people of lifelong pain. I watched my grandmother collapse and then recover after my father held her and whispered song lyrics to her. I've also seen it fail. One member of our community had cataracts for many years, which easily could have been treated by an eye surgeon. But she was determined to treat them through her faith. As the years progressed, she slowly went blind.

What separates one from the other? How can one person get up and walk while the one next to her stays trapped in a wheelchair, crushed under the pain of arthritis? It's a question scientists have been wondering about from the second the placebo effect was described, and they have been clamoring for an answer ever since placebos became the gatekeepers of modern medicine.

It's a mystery at least one scientist thinks she just might have cracked.

CHAPTER THREE

Hunting *the* Mysterious Placebo Responder

I would rather know the person who has the disease than the disease the person has.

—Hippocrates

IN 2003, MIKE PAULETICH, THEN 42, started noticing that something strange was happening with his hands. It was subtle at first; he couldn't brush his teeth at the same speed as he had before. Pretty soon he noticed that his aim had trailed off as well. He coached his son's baseball team, and he found most of his throws going either 10 feet over the kid's head or straight into the dirt at his player's feet. He went to a neurologist, suspecting carpal tunnel syndrome. But when the test results came in, the news was very different. He had early onset Parkinson's disease. He could expect to be in a wheelchair in 10 years and probably unable to feed himself.

Parkinson's is a degenerative disease that has no cure and cannot be reversed. About all a patient can hope for is to stave off its effects as long as possible. Pauletich was devastated. A devoted family man and athlete, he realized that his brain would slowly rob him of access to his body and perhaps eventually rob his family of its father. For the next 10 years, he did what so many others in his condition have done: experiment with an unending line of drugs and scour the literature for experimental trials that were seeking patients. He didn't deteriorate as much as his doctor predicted, but the disease took its toll; he struggled with depression and hopelessness as talking and writing became ever harder.

In 2011, Pauletich finally found what he was looking for. A small biotech firm called Ceregene was experimenting with a new type of gene therapy. Essentially, it was targeting specific neurons with a protein called neurturin, which helps regulate brain cells, especially early in life. The idea was that this protein, if delivered to the right cells, could get them back on track and producing dopamine (remember that dopamine reduction is a cause of Parkinson's). It was a simple matter of drilling into a patient's head and delivering the protein directly. The problem was that so far it hadn't worked. Ceregene had tried the technique once before, in 2006, with a limited human trial that was ultimately unsuccessful. Gene therapy—the notion that you can tinker directly with the genes of ailing human cells—has held tremendous promise for many years. But like stem cell therapy, cold fusion, and reboots of *The Muppet Show*, it's beginning to look like a breakthrough that's never going to happen.

After careful examination, Ceregene decided that three flaws in the study had caused its previous failure. First, it had been too short. One year wasn't enough time to see the improvement the company was sure was in store for the patients. The patients who signed up first, and thus had been observed for longer than a year, seemed to do better than the newcomers did. Second, the neurturin didn't seem to be getting to the right part of the brain. They had treated a structure deep in the brain called the putamen, hoping it would transmit the protein to an even deeper part, the substantia nigra. But the drug didn't seem to make the journey. And last, the patients weren't meant to know which of them got the real treatment and which of them received a sham surgery, but many of them had deduced it by talking with other patients on social media.

The sham surgery was the placebo control. The patients who got it would receive the same treatment as those getting the real surgery; the only difference was that their surgeon would not drill all the way into their brains, but just far enough into the skull to create a convincing divot. This may seem cruel to you and me, but Parkinson's is a devious disease. One of the reasons it has been so hard to cure is that it seems to respond more to placebo treatments than other degenerative brain ailments do.

The study was double-blind, meaning neither the patients nor the doctors knew who got which surgery. But the team suspected that the patients had contacted one another and compared notes. Twitter and Facebook are loaded with patient groups where people can find each other and discuss effects and side effects. If a patient with only mild side effects reads that other people are reacting strongly to a treatment, she might deduce that she's in the placebo group. Yes, you read that right. People in a placebo group can experience side effects, occasionally so severe that they drop out of the study.

This was about the time that Pauletich found Ceregene. Two years after the initial experiment, the company's back was against the wall. Ceregene suspected it had something that could halt Parkinson's in its tracks and improve the lives of some seven million people globally. But trials like these are expensive. One more miss would put the company into bankruptcy. In the end, Ceregene decided to go for it and made exactly the kind of bold move that has always come before science's greatest discoveries.

Kathleen Poston was one of the researchers on the project and Pauletich's doctor. A Parkinson's specialist at Stanford University, Poston is a vivacious woman with strong features, a round face, and long brown hair. Every day, she said, she sees the devastating effects of Parkinson's and has dedicated her life to helping patients any way she can.

According to Poston, Ceregene had reason to be optimistic. The new study would use cutting-edge techniques involving a harmless virus that would carry the neurturin directly to a deeper part of the brain. This time the study would run for 18 to 24 months. Placebo effects are the biggest problems bedeviling Parkinson's work, but they are usually short-lived; no one could imagine them persisting for more than a year. And subjects would be counseled not to use social media to contact one another.

They chose 51 subjects for the experiment, all with serious late-stage Parkinson's disease. Pauletich, 10 years into his diagnosis, was one of them. He didn't seem as sick as the others, but Poston had lobbied to bring him on. Twenty-four people got the real surgery, and 27 got a sham surgery involving all the same preparation as the real surgery—shaving the head, anesthesia, drilling, and regular checkups afterward. Four of them were Poston's patients, but none of the patients' doctors knew who had received the real treatment. That said, a doctor can often tell. Subtle side effects and certain responses are clearly the work of an active therapy. And with a patient like Pauletich, it wasn't even subtle.

"There were times when I would be on business calls before the surgery and the client would hang up . . . and call the salesperson back and say, 'You know, I appreciate Mike's at a conference in Vegas, but does he have to come to the calls drunk? Because he's slurring his words," Pauletich told me. "Within a few weeks [of the surgery] that cleared up quite a bit, and it just got better and better over time. My handwriting got better. My performance on tests was quicker, and all around I was feeling like, wow, I finally found a drug that worked."

In the year and a half after the surgery, Pauletich's life turned around. He was able to work and carry on his life much as he had before his diagnosis. His mood lifted and his mobility increased. He started working out and ran a triathlon; he even went heli-skiing with his son. Poston was ecstatic: "In my head I kept thinking, 'If we finally have found something that slows disease progression, then that's a game changer,'" she said.

Another patient of Poston's had failed to improve and had even gotten worse with treatment, experiencing more tremors and an increased feeling of being trapped in his own body. Clearly this patient had received the sham surgery. And sad as that may seem, it was vital to contrast against Pauletich's amazing strides. Better yet, the trial's promise had broader implications beyond Parkinson's. A success like this could revitalize gene-therapy research in a dozen other diseases. It was the kind of moment every scientist dreams of: the chance to really help people. In the fall of 2014, the team joined a conference call to learn Ceregene's official results. But from the first moment, Poston knew something was wrong.

"There was just this heaviness. This weight," she said. "I've been on these conference calls before when they announce the results. And you can tell the moment you dial in whether it's a positive or negative study, just by that weight."

The study had failed. There was no statistical difference between those who had received the treatment and those who had received the sham surgery. By the time it published its paper on the study a few months later, Ceregene had been acquired by another company, its research on indefinite hold, and the breakthrough in gene therapy for countless diseases once again stymied.

After the call, Poston got the details of the study, and what she saw stopped her cold. Pauletich had been in the placebo group.

● ● ●

The problem of placebo responders is the central challenge to modern medicine. The placebo response not only has the power to kill a proposed drug that doesn't work; it also has the power to block one that does. From start to finish, a single prescription drug costs more than $2.5 billion to bring to market. It's impossible to know exactly how many drugs never come to market every year in America because of the high placebo response. That information is the property of private companies, but people around the industry often say it's about half, possibly as much as three-quarters. And while we can't know what drugs are failing, it's a good bet that many are targeting pain, depression, and stomach discomfort—all highly placebo responsive and, when they make it through drug trials, reaching the largest markets for patients. At least a third of the world's top 10 blockbuster drugs are aimed at placebo-responsive conditions like pain and arthritis, asthma, and Crohn's disease.[7]

And there are sham surgeries like the one that Pauletich received. Because of the high placebo responses among Parkinson's patients, sham surgeries have become almost required in recent years to test the efficacy of any experimental therapy or drug aimed at this disease. Just to give you a sense of what this looks like, the primary measurement of Parkinson's improvement is a set of mobility and flexibility tests called the Unified Parkinson's Disease Rating Scale. Studies suggest that placebo pills have the power to give patients as much as 10 percent more mobility, while a sham surgery can provide up to 25 percent more mobility. In other words, surgery is psychologically more powerful than a pill. A common joke among researchers is that the greatest advance in Parkinson's medicine over the past decade has been the sham surgery.

All this is to say that the placebo effect is a multibillion-dollar problem for the drug industry and certainly keeps good drugs from getting to market. Take a depression drug like Prozac. The development of Prozac was bedeviled by high placebo rates that made it hard

---

7 Interestingly, Crohn's responds better to placebos taken over longer periods of time, which is counterintuitive if placebos are indeed short-lived.

to tell if it worked. It obviously made it to your pharmacist's shelf, but nowadays many scientists say it is not effective enough to outperform placebos. (It's still on the market because once a drug clears the FDA, it cannot be recalled just because the placebo effect gets stronger.) There are two possible reasons for this. One, the expectation for relief from Prozac has grown. Today Prozac (and drugs like it) is a household name, and everyone knows what to expect when they take it. Thus the expectation—and the placebo effect—is higher than it was back in 1987, when it was cleared by the FDA. On the other hand, there is some evidence that placebo effects are going up across the board, though the reasons for this aren't clear.

But imagine if before Ceregene even started the trial it could have eliminated all the people who were going to have a placebo response—not just those in the placebo group but also those who received the real treatment. (Remember, just because a person is getting an active drug doesn't mean he can't experience a placebo effect.) What if there was some evidence that certain people were more likely to respond to a placebo than others, and they could be identified and excluded from experiments? Suddenly, not only would drugs be cheaper to test but also you would know right away whether they worked.

The World War II doctor and placebo pioneer Henry Beecher himself—father of the placebo study—was among the first to test this hypothesis, reasoning that perhaps people who frequently go to church are more likely to be swayed by the authority of a doctor. Other researchers thought suggestibility might be related to intelligence or education or age or gender. Perhaps the severity of the disease played a role. People tried Rorschach tests to find a link. One unpleasant 1961 paper written in Louisiana declared that black people were particularly vulnerable to placebos, according to one unaffiliated scientist, because of a "prevalent attitude amongst the negroes to please their doctor." I wish I could say such attitudes are a thing of the past, but study after study has shown that even today white medical professionals rate black patients' pain lower than that of other whites. One study even showed that black kids with appendicitis are significantly less likely to get pain drugs in the ER compared with white kids.

Naturally, none of these ideas panned out under scientific scrutiny. And after Senator Kefauver's 1962 Drug Efficacy Amendment requiring that every drug receive a Phase III placebo-controlled trial (meaning, be given to big groups of people to evaluate its safety and effectiveness), drugs were becoming harder and harder to create.

So scientists began looking for other cues—this time not along racial or gender lines, but psychological ones. That led to a link between placebo and "acquiescence," or the propensity to agree with people. Another link appeared with people who are hypnotizable, and another with people whose minds tend to wander a lot. Children were often found to be especially placebo prone. A 1983 study showed that insomniacs who were "more attentive to internal bodily processes" were more likely to experience placebo responses than others. A series of bizarre experiments with nonalcoholic beer in the 1980s suggested that people at risk for alcoholism were less likely to have placebo responses. In the past couple of decades, scientists have shifted to a theory called dispositional optimism, or the measure of how glass-half-full you are as a possible measure of how placebo prone you are.

Some of these theories—notably that hypnotizable people are more placebo prone—stuck around, but most ended up being dead-ends. And none were truly replicable, a requirement for any scientific finding. It seems that a person might respond to one placebo today but not tomorrow, and then to a different one the day after that, with no rhyme or reason. Try to limit the number of responders, such as by giving everybody in the trial a placebo for the first few weeks and then culling out the responders, and new placebo responders who didn't respond the first time just took their place. Then there are other placebo-like effects that confuse the issue—for example, the Hawthorne effect, which causes people to feel better just because someone is studying them. Or there are people who feel better simply because the disease went away naturally. Others don't feel better but say they do because it's what the physician wants to hear.

Clearly, screening for placebo responsiveness is no simple matter. Suggestibility, for all its power and ubiquitousness, can be incredibly elusive.

"Dealing with expectation is very tricky. Do you really think that expectation is a stable phenomenon? Doesn't it change every five minutes? We're dealing with very imprecise measuring of a very imprecise phenomenon. And a lot of it's non-conscious," says Ted Kaptchuk, the pioneering Harvard placebo researcher. "There is a phenomenon here. But capturing it has not been easy."

Whether it's because of a higher level of expectation on the part of patients or changes in the diseases of people taking the drugs, one of the greatest challenges in medicine today is to create a new drug for pain, depression, anxiety, or upset stomachs. And at roughly two billion dollars per medication, companies can't afford to spend years on a depression or a pain cure only to see it go down in flames because of a high placebo response. Yet over the past six decades the pharmaceutical industry has slowly lost interest in identifying the elusive placebo responder, leaving the quest to scientists in the cash-strapped halls of academia to pursue. By 2012, it was time for something new.

• • •

Though I've spent a lot of time talking to scientists, the first time I meet Kathryn Hall near her office at Harvard University, I have to say she baffles me. Her long hair, streaked with gray and twisted into dreadlocks, is pulled back from her face. She is uncommonly expressive, and her voice is a forceful alto with a hint of a Jamaican accent. When she says she once dabbled in a Reiki-like form of aura cleansing and even cured herself of carpal tunnel syndrome through acupuncture I categorize her as a well-meaning hippie on a quest to undermine the big bad pharmaceutical industry. Then she launches into a monologue about the wonders of drugmaking and the importance of modern pharmaceuticals that sounds more Genentech than it does Woodstock.

Hall says she decided to study placebos to make drugs better, not to undermine them. She understands why pharmaceutical companies lost interest in studying placebos. For too long they were just too amorphous, too psychological. Scientists lacked tangible mechanisms to examine—something they could pull apart and study. This talk of brain chemicals is fine, but a drug company needs a gene pathway, not some fluffy conversation about expectation and dispositional optimism. They need something to explain why the brain acts the way it does.

Hall knew that dopamine is important in placebo responses, so she put together a list of all the gene pathways that seemed to relate to dopamine and opioids. She needed something big, something tied to reward systems, something with a lot of research behind it. One gene on the list stood out: catechol-O-methyltransferase, or *COMT*. The *COMT* gene codes for an enzyme in the brain, also called *COMT*. It's one of the best-studied brain pathways in the world and may be the most fascinating thing I have ever discovered as a science writer. Bear with me while I explain it. I promise the payoff will be worth it.

Here's how it works. We learned about dopamine and the enormous power that it wields in the body. As awesome as it may be for body movement and good moods, it's always possible to have too much of a good thing. Our brains need a mechanism to sweep up the bits we don't need—the extra dopamine molecules floating around our skulls that aren't doing anything useful. That's *COMT*. I like to think of it as little Pac-Men that go around neutralizing dopamine molecules. They don't technically destroy dopamine, but they do oxidize it, thus changing it forever and taking it out of commission for much of its work.

"Dopamine is so central to who we are. Anything that modifies dopamine is going to modify a lot of things," Hall says. "If you mess around with a critical kind of player like *COMT,* then you are going to affect a lot of different systems."

Like all enzymes, *COMT* is horribly long and complicated, with lots of moving parts. But it turns out that this enzyme has one spot, one tiny gear within its machinery that essentially defines how well it works. Depending on your genetics, this crucial portion of the enzyme can be one of two types: valine (val) or methionine (met). Now, if this massive molecule happens to have valine in that one spot, the enzyme does its job like a good soldier, seeking out every available dopamine molecule and neutralizing it. Your brain has little excess dopamine and runs efficiently, like a Swiss watch. On the other hand, if the enzyme has methionine in that one spot, it is far less effective. In other words, a valine-laced enzyme is captain of her volleyball team while taking night school courses and holding down three jobs. A methionine *COMT* enzyme, meanwhile, is the kind of molecule who spends all his time doing bong rips and playing Grand Theft Auto in his mom's basement.

As a result, there is a lot of extra dopamine in those brains with methionine. Now, it turns out that this crucial valine/methionine component in *COMT* enzymes is determined by a single gene—in fact, just a single rung on the DNA ladder. If you remember your high school genetics, you will recall that every trait in your body is a combination of contributions from each of your parents. If both your parents have blue eyes (b), you will too (bb).[8] If one of your folks gives you a brown-eye gene (B) and the other a blue-eye one (b), your eyes

---

8 Eye color actually depends on a number of genes, but I use it as an example here because it's easy and because almost no trait in our genomes except *COMT* hinges on only a single rung of DNA.

will be brown (Bb) because brown is dominant. If your mate has blue eyes, your kids have a 50 percent chance of having blue eyes, depending on which "b" you end up giving them.

COMT works exactly the same way. Most of us have a combination of valine and methionine, meaning we have some lazy enzymes and some industrious ones. We are *val/mets*, and we aren't nearly as interesting as the other two groups. The second possibility is that a person gets two valine genes from her parents and her enzymes pull extra shifts to keep her brain clean of dopamine. She is called a *val/val*. The last is the fellow who gets two methionine genes and has *COMT* enzymes that get off the couch only when they run out of Cheetos and beer. This person has lots of extra dopamine floating around, looking for a place to be of use while the janitors meant to clean them up look for a good place to hang a hammock and take a nap. He's a *met/met*.

The world is made up of about half val/mets, one-quarter val/vals, and one-quarter met/mets. The hardworking val/val enzymes are three or four times more active than the met/mets. Few single genes in our bodies have so much power in determining how our brains operate. Because dopamine is such a crucial chemical in the brain, changes in an enzyme that moderates it can have a huge effect on the way we think and act. *COMT* has been linked to just about everything from jaw pain to insomnia to schizophrenia. It may also be involved in bipolar disorder.

It's a lot to keep in mind, I know. Here's a handy chart to check back on as you read:

val/val	all industrious enzymes (little excess dopamine)	25% of population
met/me	all lazy enzymes (lots of excess dopamine)	25% of population
val/met	combination of lazy and industrious enzymes	50% of population

One study found that val/val kids who had traumatic life experiences were more likely to be aggressive than met/mets, whereas the reverse was true of kids who did not have these experiences. Another found that val/vals are more susceptible to gambling addiction, and some say they perform mental tasks better under pressure but struggle to maintain focus in daily life. Met/mets may be vulnerable to eating disorders and are more sensitive to pain. Lots of things have been said about the behavior of met/mets over the years (no doubt by val/vals, who dominate the halls of science laboratories), but one of the most consistent is that they tend to rate experiences as more pleasurable than val/vals do. Have you ever been to a movie with a group of friends and one of them is just a little too effusive?

"Oh my God, that was the BEST MOVIE EVER! Scarlett Johansson is amazing, and the Hulk is just an enormous badass!" he says. This is classic met/met. With so much extra dopamine, met/mets tend to be effusive and emotive, and they rate their experiences more intensely than their cohorts do. Then there's that other friend who walks out of the theater scratching her head. "I dunno. The plot was way more complicated than it had to be, and Captain America was awful. And what was the deal with all the aliens?" Textbook val/val. Her efficient *COMT* enzymes have taken all the unneeded dopamine out of the mix and left her very matter-of-fact.

These generalizations, of course, are meant to describe large groups of people, not individuals. A thousand met/mets will be more effusive on average than a thousand val/vals but not all met/mets are balls of emotion and not all val/vals are sticks-in-the-mud. Furthermore, scientists are less interested in using this sort of genetic theory to explain why a person acts a certain way and more in understanding the relationship between brain chemicals and behavior. (Nevertheless, after spending a lot of time with the literature, I began to believe I could spot a *COMT* genotype a mile away. Barack Obama? Total val/

val. Oprah Winfrey, met/met; German chancellor Angela Merkel, val/val; Tom Cruise, met/met.)

A few years ago, Hall concocted an experiment to pair *COMT* genes with placebos. First she enrolled 262 patients with irritable bowel syndrome (which is highly placebo prone) into an experimental treatment involving acupuncture. Hall selected patients with either moderate or severe cases of IBS and split them up into three groups. One group was put on a waiting list and basically got nothing: a true control group. The other two were told they would have acupuncture. Everyone in the group got fake acupuncture—needles that look like they go into your skin but actually don't. Hall wasn't interested in whether it worked or not. The point was that half the patients got treatment from a comforting, caring acupuncturist while the others got a rather cold, uncaring one.

What she found was startling. As expected, regardless of their genes, the people on the waiting list stayed about the same. Meanwhile, met/mets with the uncaring doctor did better than the val/vals, but just barely. The val/vals who got the caring doctor did about as well as the val/vals who got the uncaring doctor and all the people on the waiting list. But the val/mets who got the nice doctor did about five times better. And the results of the met/mets who got the caring doctor went through the roof. Clearly, a few kind words meant something totally different to one genotype than it did to all the others. For the first time, Hall had sliced off placebo responders into a measurable group. Met/mets— those people who were born with lazy enzymes and a little too much dopamine in their systems—were more prone to placebo responses.

With a tool like this, suddenly everything about placebos seemed to make sense. My wife—a met/met if ever there was one—is prone to all kinds of suggestion and placebos. Tom Cruise—as I said before, an obvious met/met—claims to have experienced healing powers within the Church of Scientology. By the time I finished Hall's paper

I was wondering if perhaps I could persuade someone to genotype the entire Christian Science Church to see how many are met/mets.

The concept makes great evolutionary sense as well. Just as it's good to have some members of a population who are stronger, faster, or smarter than others, it's probably good to have varying levels of suggestibility. Some people need to be clear-eyed and unmoved, like the val/vals. But nature thrives on variety and has given us an equal number of suggestible people who have an extraordinary genetic tool that allows them to heal themselves. For a couple of years, I thought maybe science had found a simple answer to the question of who responds to placebos. *COMT* was, in essence, the placebo gene. But in 2015, Hall and fellow Harvard researcher Ted Kaptchuk followed up with another paper that identified not just dopamine but a whole suite of brain chemicals that might play roles in various placebo responses.

You see, although the *COMT* gene plays an outsize role in the creation of the *COMT* enzyme, it's not the *only* gene that does so. Several other genes that help build the enzyme can boost or cripple its performance, to say nothing of all the other genes in your body that affect dopamine. Plus, just as a blueprint doesn't always match the building, so DNA doesn't always match the part of your body that it codes for. Changes can happen along the way.

Also, *COMT* doesn't just pick on dopamine; it also goes after epinephrine and norepinephrine, neurotransmitters that are key to regulating adrenaline, cardiac function, and our response to stress. Epinephrine is also related to heart disease, hypertension, triglyceride levels, and hemoglobin. In one study, Hall found that met/mets taking placebos had poorer outcomes for heart problems than those who took aspirin, which makes sense, since aspirin is a proven heart medication. She also found that aspirin affects heart disease differently in met/mets and val/vals.

And then there are the competitors. *COMT,* it turns out, isn't alone in regulating dopamine. Several other genes play a role in different parts of the body and different parts of the chemical's life span. And there are other brain chemicals that have their own agenda when it comes to placebo and expectation. There's serotonin and opioids and, as I mentioned before, even naturally occurring cannabinoids.[9] If you are a placebo responder in dopamine but not in serotonin, what does that mean? What if two genes that both regulate dopamine are diametrically opposed to each other?

I want to know where I stand in all this, so I take a few minutes to spit into a little plastic vial and mail it to the genetic analysis company 23andMe. After a couple of weeks, I get an email that grants me access to my entire genome, or at least all the genes that I'll need to assess my own placebo responsiveness. I find myself oddly conflicted. On the one hand, I want to think of myself as a val/val—calm, logical, reliable. On the other hand, it would be nice to have a strong proclivity to placebo responses. The truth, it turns out, is far less interesting. I'm val/met. A mix, like half the world's population. It turns out the same is true for the genes that control my cannabinoids and my MAO-A (another, weaker actor in my dopamine system), which might further inhibit my ability to experience placebo effects.

I take my genome report to Kathryn Hall, and only one of the genes she has evaluated jumps out. It's *OPRM1,* located on my sixth chromosome. It plays a role in pain reception and cravings for alcohol. That gene, Hall says, determines the chemical that coats a crucial group of opioid receptors in my brain. This is the part of my brain

---

9 Let that sink in. You were born with some of the same chemicals that help create the experience of being high. And your brain distributes them whenever it feels it's appropriate. Similarly, you have enough serotonin in your brain to stay high for hours (as anyone who's tried the drug ecstasy can tell you). It's no wonder our brains came up with so many chemical regulators—if you're not careful, you could overdose on your own brain.

that receives painkilling drugs—whether given to me by a doctor, a drug dealer, or my own brain—and codes that experience into what I then feel. If I have a chemical called aspartic acid at that key spot, it will run inefficiently and hinder my brain's ability to feel relief or elation. On the other hand, if my receptors use a chemical called asparagine, the receptors work perfectly and I experience the full flood of any drug.

This is a totally different setup than with *COMT*. The *COMT* gene determined how much of a drug I have available in my brain, while *OPRM1* determines how my brain absorbs a drug. But the results can be striking. Some studies show that people with aspartic acid are more likely to be caught up in alcoholism, and others show that those same people are more likely to respond to drugs used to help alcoholics stop drinking. Meanwhile, those with asparagine on their receptors are more likely to feel pain relief from placebo effects.

Despite being an utter failure at placebo genetics, my genetic test shows that my opioid receptors are covered in the highly efficient, brain-soothing asparagine. Could it be that my lack of extra dopamine keeps me from experiencing the powerful placebo responses that some other people do? But when I do experience a placebo response—at least with pain—it comes across loud and clear? That would explain my time in Luana Colloca's torture chair.

"That's really interesting," Hall says, when I tell her about my experience getting shocked at NIH. She pauses. "We've never thought this through in this way."

It seems that, after just a couple of hours and a few cups of tea, we're already coming up against the limits of the science as we currently understand it. For one thing, we don't have a full list of all the chemicals involved in placebo responses, and we don't know how they interact. Which ones are more important? Which ones are holding others back, and which are further enhancing the effects? But more important, the studies that Hall relies on are based on averages and large numbers of people. Saying that a healthy percentage of met/mets have one reaction to fake acupuncture or that a slice of the asparagine people have another reaction to saline injections is not the same as saying what is happening in my actual brain as I visit the homeopath's office.

The nice thing about this model, though, is that for the first time we have an explanation for the mysterious placebo responder that isn't mysterious. It's a crack in the wall that suggests a reason why some people seem to respond to one placebo and not another, why the placebo response can seem so clear in one person and not in another, and why it seems vaguely related to personality and at the same time totally divorced from it. Homeopathy patients, Christian Scientists, TCM—suddenly all these phenomena make more sense. What if the reason some people experience such relief from prayer healing and unproven therapies while others don't is that they simply have different genetic maps for self-medication?

"Something is going on," says Kaptchuk, who was Hall's mentor and co-authored her work. "I think Kathryn Hall may have found the glimmer of a possibility of the Holy Grail."

For her part, Hall is far less interested in jumping to conclusions than I am. She says that, if anything, her work shows that you don't really know much about a test subject until you take her genetic data. Trying out a new drug to treat addiction? Be sure you know how your subjects uptake opioids. Want to try a new pain med? Maybe you should check their COMT genes first. From here on out, she explains, no one should be doing placebo research, or really any pharmaceutical testing, without first collecting some information about what genes might be throwing wrenches into the works. And along the way, we may find the key to a whole new type of medicine, personalized and tailored to people's specific strengths and weaknesses. This promises to be a revolutionary development in the way medicine is delivered to individuals and could potentially give us more options and cheaper drugs, as we will learn next.

• • •

If you are a pharmaceutical company testing a drug against a placebo, all you want to know is whether a person responded or not. But the real story—the important one—is the details. In a war, there are thousands of skirmishes and unintended consequences that do not remotely reflect the ultimate outcome. In the same way, teasing apart the vast, complicated set of reactions that happen in our bodies when we are having a placebo response is far more interesting than whether the placebo worked or not. In other words, the nuances are the fun parts—and the useful ones.

Still, there are plenty of people who would say that knowing whether a person will respond to a placebo in advance would be an incredibly powerful tool for making better drugs. That's certainly what former pharmaceutical executive Gunther Winkler hopes. For 23 years he was deep in the trenches of drug development, primarily for the massive biotech company Biogen, which makes hundreds of drugs that affect the brain, blood, and immune system. His work was creating and shepherding new drugs through the labyrinthine process of development and FDA certification. Every year, a company like Biogen sees many drugs that work great on rats. But they can choose only one or two to take to the next level, since the most difficult and expensive part of creating a drug is recruiting and testing human patients in bigger studies. Winkler says each person enrolled in an experiment ends up costing the company a shocking $30,000, including time and resources. Considering that even a minimal "proof of concept" study—to prove that a drug is even worth the effort of testing—requires hundreds of subjects, costs can accumulate quickly. This, he says, is one of the fundamental problems in modern drugmaking. "The one thing that always came back to me was, drug development is too expensive; drug development takes too long," he says.

At first glance, Winkler seems like the prototypical biotech executive—shaved head, expensive business casual wear, and a polished message about his company. But he is also genuinely passionate about the potential of drugmakers to help ease the suffering of disease. After a successful career as a pharmaceutical executive and now in his 50s, he has every right to buy an island somewhere in the South Pacific and take up spearfishing. But instead he wants to dedicate the rest of his life to making drugs more effective and efficient. If there was such a thing as a corporate pharmaceutical idealist, it would be Gunther Winkler.

When he first heard about Hall's work with *COMT* genes, like me, a light went off in his head and his pulse started racing. Winkler had worked on a variety of drugs to alleviate numerous medical conditions at Biogen, but the one thing that linked them all together was the placebo response. For instance, he had worked on a drug aimed at treating psoriasis, an itchy and uncomfortable skin condition caused by an autoimmune deficiency. Psoriasis patients are highly susceptible to placebos. According to Winkler, these psoriasis placebo effects seemed dependent on psychology and mood. If a suffering patient goes on vacation or removes a stressor from his life, the discomfort tends to evaporate. Winkler says he could spend decades chasing down each condition like psoriasis and trying to streamline the process of creating drugs for them. But by eliminating placebo responders, he could hit them all at once.

The higher the placebo response to a given drug, the more people you need in the study to prove that the drug isn't capitalizing on that placebo response. But if you could somehow exclude met/mets from a trial and bring down the placebo response, you could dramatically lower that number required to reach statistical significance—leaving aside for now the ethical dilemma here. Imagine a small drug trial with a 44 percent placebo response. Normally, Winkler says, you need more than 360 patients to be sure the results weren't distorted by placebo responses. But if you could get the placebo responders down to 24 percent, you would need a minimum of 72 subjects to prove whether the drug was effective or not.

Would this work in the real world? Unlike most academics, Winkler's years of experience in the pharmaceutical industry give him contacts and access to massive data sets from previous drug trials—data representing hundreds of thousands of actual patients that academics would drool over but that are proprietary to the company.

Winkler says that he approached one company (he declined to mention its name) and asked to apply the met/met screen to the results of one of its depression-drug trials. The drug it was testing (he also declined to mention its name) had eventually passed FDA trials but naturally had been extremely expensive (he declined to say how expensive). But when this company went back through its data and screened out met/mets, it found, lo and behold, the *COMT* gene would have predicted who was going to eventually respond to the placebos in the trial. All because of a single rung on a single strand of DNA.

Faster than you can say IPO, Winkler patented the met/met screen, and in late 2013 created a new company called Biometheus, which essentially offers to screen a company's trial participants for met/mets. Even if such a screen uncovers only a fraction of the actual responders, it could offer huge savings for drugmakers. At first he hopes to sell his technique to biotech companies, but eventually he wants to see them adopt it as their own.

After thousands of years, the placebo response isn't going anywhere. It's hardwired into who we are on a neurochemical level. And after decades of searching for the perfect placebo responder, scientists have finally admitted that they may never be able to separate him or her from the rest of humanity. But using our genetic information, they may have the first ever tool to start trying. Still, there is one problem. If the screening works, the drugs that come out of this process may be certified only for use by people with val/val or val/met genotypes. On the one hand, this would be exciting, since they would be among the first gene-specific drugs to hit the market and the first therapies to be specifically tailored to our genes. Imagine you had, say, persistent leg pain that just wasn't going away with any of the drugs you were prescribed. Eventually a doctor takes a sample of your DNA, learns you are a val/val, and prescribes a new pain med that otherwise would have been tossed on the junk heap of failed drugs.

But what about all those poor met/mets out there? Don't they deserve effective therapies too? Hall and Gunther point out that met/mets respond well to both placebos and regular drugs. It's just that their brain chemistry has the bonus of supercharging their response. All things considered, they are actually the most fortunate members of the population. They can take the drug and they will respond at a higher level than the recalcitrant val/vals. Or, if they decide that conventional medicine isn't their thing, they can try acupuncture, homeopathy, or faith healing and perhaps do just as well—whereas on a val/val, those treatments are more likely to fall flat.

The great thing about these findings is that it may not matter if met/mets are aware of their predisposition. As we've learned, many placebo responses seem to dwell outside our conscious thought, so it makes no difference whether we know we're taking a placebo or whether we have particularly responsive placebo genes.

Imagine a world in which a doctor takes a sample of your blood and, while you sit in the waiting room reading *Surfer* magazine, runs an analysis of your *COMT* gene. And when you get back in the office, she says, "I have a list of drugs for you to try to alleviate your arthritis.

And in case those don't work, well, I've looked at your genome, and I have the name of a really good brujo you can try."

Early scientists considered people who responded to placebo medicine to be somehow impure, naive, soft. But they may be the lucky ones. They are the ones who can take both conventional medicines and select from a wild menagerie of placebos that tap into their beliefs and their expectations and allow their minds to cure themselves. Perhaps permanently. Who are these people? We don't know yet. But sitting in a Berkeley, California, café in February 2016, I learn who they might be from the Parkinson's patient who is their poster child.

• • •

Mike Pauletich's experience with Ceregene did indeed change his life, though not in the way he had initially expected. "It really was a gut punch," he says of the moment when he learned that the miracle cure he had received was nothing but a placebo. "It took a while to process."

Certainly, it could have dragged him down. Before the surgery, he was depressed and not exercising, and his marriage was suffering. It would have been easy to go right back to that. But in that moment Pauletich made a decision. He didn't let this disease dictate how his life would go. Sure his miracle drug was nothing but an endogenous bodily response to expectation. But it had come from within himself, and he had the power to keep it going. He decided to take control of his own disease. Three years since his sham brain surgery, he hasn't seen any kind of drop-off in his health or mobility and in fact feels like he has a whole new lease on life.

"It's not a death sentence," he says. "It's a call to action: to take care of yourself, to do the things that you need to do to stay healthy."

So what happened to Pauletich? It's a question that scientists will continue to puzzle over for years to come. Certainly his experience is among the longest placebo responses ever recorded. Perhaps all he needed was a reason to get more exercise or just break the funk he was in. But what if the suggestion that he'd undergone a new, miraculous surgery somehow changed the functioning of his brain? And what if this extended placebo response over the course of two years helped rewire his brain in some permanent way? What if expectation was the trigger that allowed his brain to identify a problem and fix it on its own?

When he was first diagnosed, Pauletich's worst fear was that he wouldn't get to see his son grow up or participate in his son's life. To throw a baseball with him or show him the world. But when I talked to him, he was preparing for a ski adventure with his son, and the two of them were planning to hike in Yosemite together. This was not the result of positive thinking or some meaningless platitude from one of a thousand books that promise miracle cures. Mike Pauletich had tapped into the very basic functioning of his own brain and came out the other side a better man.

"It's not 'telling yourself.' You can't fool yourself. You have to *believe* that you have control over it. That the disease is not going to take control of you, that you are going to take control of it," he says. "It's a difference between belief and hope. At some point there's a switch between 'I hope I'm going to get better' and 'I know I can defeat this.' "

We are just beginning to understand that the power of suggestibility can be an incredible tool to cure us of our worst diseases. When it comes to the power of the mind to change the body, the easiest condition to study so far has been pain. But stories like Mike Pauletich's open a window onto a larger world of placebo responders who may actually hold keys to a wide array of long-term health benefits. We know that placebo responses are real, measurable neurochemical events in the brain. We know a little about the ways that shamans and physicians have harnessed them over the centuries. And we know that different placebo responses are controlled by both different brain pathways and different genetics, which explains why people seem to experience them in such diverse ways.

But do the same rules apply to all placebos? Are there placebo responses that we have yet to discover? For instance, cancer historically has not responded well to placebo treatments, yet plenty of dubious treatments have claimed to cure the disease. Are they all hokum, or is there perhaps some yet-to-be-discovered mechanism by which the mind can affect a cancerous tumor?

There is a lot about expectation and the mind that we just don't understand yet. How much of it is chemical and how much is a statistical anomaly or self-delusion on the part of the patient? Certainly placebos enhance the effect of a drug, but do they also interact with a drug—just as one would expect when you mix two chemicals inside the human body?

Most important, if there was ever truly a way to separate placebo responders from the rest of society—either by personality or brain scans or genetics—what would we do with that information? Bar them from all drug trials? If we did that, wouldn't we have to bar them from taking the drugs that came out of such trials? Placebo research promises to open the a path to some of the first truly personalized medicine on Earth. But will that medicine prove an inspiring beacon of inclusion or a will it be just another way to classify and exclude people?

The placebo effect is an elegant and fascinating phenomenon that beckons us to dig deeper into its mysteries. It is at the same time broadly significant and deeply personal. It reaches to the earliest days of recorded history and out to a new, gleaming future. And mastering it has the potential to give each of us a blueprint for mastering our own health.

But as exciting as placebo research may be, it's only one part of the power of suggestibility in our lives. In the next chapters we'll learn about other tricks of the mind and the glimpses they give us into our remarkable, suggestible brains.

PART TWO

Your Mind's Parlor Tricks

CHAPTER FOUR

The Dark Side *of* Suggestion

The only thing we have to fear is fear itself.

—Franklin Delano Roosevelt

IN 1886, A PHYSICIAN NAMED JOHN MACKENZIE was treating a woman with a serious case of hay fever and accompanying asthma. He noted that she was "stout" and "well nourished," with light hair, brown eyes, and a fair complexion. He also noted, a little unsympathetically, that she was "physically weak" and had a "nervous temperament," which might have been her personality or might have been due to a brutal-sounding uterine dysfunction she experienced after the birth of her first child. Furthermore, according to Mackenzie, this nervousness ran through her family, which was riddled with allergies, asthma, headaches, scarlet fever, and neuralgia (a poorly defined and mysterious pain condition originating in the nerves and usually limited to one region of the body). Reading between the lines, we can surmise that the good doctor wasn't convinced that his patient's condition was fully authentic. So he performed an experiment. He put a rose in his office the next time she came in. As soon as she saw it, she had a powerful allergic reaction that brought on an asthma attack.

This might have qualified as torture were it not for the fact that the flower was artificial. Psychologists and allergy researchers ever since have pondered what actually happened to this woman. Was her response real? Was her disease real?

As we've discussed, suggestibility can be a pretty good thing. It can alleviate pain, cure Parkinson's, even bring communities closer together. But don't be fooled. Holmes has his Moriarty. Spider-Man has his Venom. And the placebo has its own evil alter ego.

Welcome to the dark and frightening world of the nocebo.

Recall that *placebo* is Latin for "I shall please"; *nocebo* means "I shall harm." Think of the nocebo as the placebo's ugly, cantankerous step-brother. The one no one wants to sit next to at Thanksgiving. Just as placebos *ease* pain through brain processes, nocebos *cause* it. Like placebos, nocebos can be induced in the laboratory through decep-tion. And like placebos, they tend to track alongside dopamine and opioid systems, affecting conditions like pain, nausea, depression, and anxiety. Except nocebos make those conditions worse, not better.

Nocebos can be found in almost all forms of disease. The difference is that (in the absence of horrible breaches of patients' rights) there's really only one way to study nocebos in a controlled environment: via pain. Imagine that every time a rat hears a bell, it gets an electric shock. Bell, shock. Bell, shock. Then eventually it just hears the bell; there's no shock. The rat will react just as if it had been shocked. Arguably, it may even feel the pain of a shock. That, at its most naked essence, is the nocebo response. But humans don't need conditioning the way rats do. Just a couple of words will do the trick.

The case of the woman and the rose is one of the earliest docu-mented examples of the nocebo effect, though the experiment took place long before the word had been coined. Once you know what to look for, you'll start to see nocebos everywhere. In fact, many of the studies we've explored so far have incorporated some element of nocebo research. For instance, in the late 1990s, around the same time scientists were blocking placebo effects using drugs like naloxone, the Italian neuroscientist Fabrizio Benedetti ran a similar series of experiments that looked at a hormone in the body called cholecystokinin, or CCK. It's one of those jack-of-all-trades chemicals in the body. It's a key messenger in activating intestinal functions, including digestion and the release of gastric acid and bile, and also plays a role in making you feel full after a good meal.

But if you inject CCK into someone, it causes anxiety and nausea and can induce panic attacks (which is handy for studying panic in the laboratory). In addition, CCK seems to increase pain by lessening the impact of internal opioids. This is what interested Benedetti. He set up an experiment with patients recovering from minor surgery in which he gave them a drug and told them it would make their pain worse, but it was actually just saline. (Generally a shot of salt water is considered inert—the injected version of a sugar pill. However, some scientists have argued that saline shots can cure back pain, and many doctors even use them as therapy. If this is true, it would basically invalidate every study that has used saline as a placebo.)

Sure enough, patients reported more pain with the saltwater injection. Then Benedetti blocked their brains' CCK release with another drug, much as others had done with naloxone and opioids. Except this time, the subjects felt *better* when the CCK was blocked. What opioids are for placebos, CCK is for nocebos: a mechanism giving expectation power in the body. And whereas blocking opioids killed the placebo response, and made patients feel worse, blocking CCK actually supercharged pain relief by allowing the brain's internal pharmacy to run wild.

While it's helpful to think of nocebos as placebos' evil twin, that view is not completely accurate. For instance, some studies suggest that the nocebo response is less an active process than simply the experience of pain without the buffer of a placebo response. They also seem to be easier to induce. Whereas with placebos we generally need to condition patients first, that's not necessary with nocebos. For instance, when Luana Colloca was shocking me, she had to implement two rounds of color-guided torture before she switched them up and elicited a placebo response. But if she had decided to go the opposite direction—using only the lower pain but telling me she was using the higher one—she might not have needed to condition me at all. As soon as she said, "This is really going to hurt," CCK, the stress hormone cortisol, and a healthy dose of raw panic would have kicked right in. Nocebo effects are a hell of a lot easier to create than placebo effects.

Why is this? How is it that a negative expectation can be stronger than a positive one? Think of nocebos and placebos in the brain as two different routes on Google Maps. They look similar, go to a similar place, and maybe even share a few of the same highways, but they are still totally different routes. And nocebos have all the best shortcuts. This makes logical sense, since the aversion to pain is fundamental not just to being human but also to being alive. Colloca notes that while the nocebo effect uses the same reward/expectation regions in the brain, it also taps into one more that placebos do not: fear. The hippocampus, among many other factors, plays a key role in fear conditioning and anxiety. And although it seems to be mostly absent from placebo effects, it lights up during the experience of nocebos.

If a sense of hope underlies the placebo response, then fear is at the heart of a nocebo. And fear is more powerful than you can possibly imagine. Think about news headlines. Pleasant ones certainly grab our attention: "Is Wine Good for You?" "Coffee, the New Miracle Drug," "5 Foods That Are Healthier Than You Think." But nothing gets people to click on a story like fear does. "Ebola in the Air? A Nightmare That Could Happen." "Can Wearing Your Bra Cause Cancer?" "Think Your Cat Is Plotting to Kill You? Scientists Say You Could Be Right." (All of these are real headlines. And yes, your cat is trying to kill you.)

Scary headlines simply pack a bigger punch. In 2014, even before anyone had died of Ebola in the United States, a full 25 percent of Americans were worried they or their families could contract it. Thousands of people visited doctors claiming they had signs of the virus, and 650 of those people had symptoms serious enough for their cases to be passed on to federal officials. In the end, only four people actually had the disease: two doctors who had worked in West Africa and two nurses who had treated one of them.

Consider the so-called second-year syndrome," whereby medical students become convinced they have all the diseases they are studying. Have you ever heard of it working the other way: students being convinced they're being cured by the various treatments they are studying? Of course not. We are more strongly wired for fear than for relief. Think about evolutionary theory. Who is more likely to survive: the proto human who tries a bunch of mushrooms or the cautious one who won't put them anywhere near his mouth? Sure, most of the time the first one gets a free meal while the second goes hungry. But eventually he'll eat the wrong mushroom and die. This preeminence of fear over hope is older than modern humans. We see it in animals and we see it in newborn babies who haven't developed the more advanced parts of the brain yet. Throughout the natural world, there are a few rewards for creatures that take a risk. But mostly they aren't as big as the penalties. Nature favors the cautious.

When talking about nocebos and side effects, scientists often refer to a sense of anxiety or "hypervigilance" that comes along with them. In other words, if you read that a drug you are taking causes nausea, the first thing you do is look for symptoms of nausea. If I told you that 60 percent of people who read the font in this book report feeling dizzy and tired, can you honestly say you wouldn't stop to think about whether you were maybe feeling a little tired?

One of the best places to understand the power of nocebos is in a drug trial. Take Ceregene's trial for Parkinson's disease, the one in which Mike Pauletich found out he got the placebo. According to the paper published on the study, the placebo group—Pauletich's group—had *more* side effects than those who got the real surgery. They had more instances of back pain, extremity pain, eye swelling, depression, nausea, and a whole 60 percent more headaches. How, you may wonder, can this group have had more side effects when they essentially received nothing? Can nothing have side effects?

It turns out that such phantom side effects are a relatively common phenomenon in placebo-controlled studies. In fact, many researchers are eager to showcase how safe their treatments are by noting how many fewer people experienced side effects than did those in the placebo group. But whenever I read one of these studies, I am always puzzled by how many side effects the placebo group has. Or perhaps I should call it the nocebo group.

Mostly, I wonder if this same fear and hypervigilance have the power to fundamentally alter the brain? Can nocebos become permanent? What would that even look like? Ten percent of patients in the operating room suffer from some form of continuing pain after a procedure, as do 10 percent of people recovering from accidents. Could it be that something in our brain creates a sort of metaphorical groove and falls into the habit of experiencing pain, anxiety, depression, or nausea? Could it be that chronic postoperative pain is an extended nocebo? Many diseases may be physical manifestations of fear, and understanding that may go a long way toward curing them.

But at this point, we have to broaden our definition of fear. If nocebos can transform into chronic conditions, it's probably not a conscious process. Just as placebos can happen beyond our conscious mind, so nocebos must occur in some people whether they want them or not.

But here we reach the limit of what the science of expectation can tell us. If scientists are still in the dark about long-term placebos, then they are wandering blindfolded inside a black hole wearing earplugs when it comes to chronic nocebos. I mean, how would you design an experiment causing chronic diseases in healthy human patients? That said, one group of physicians is asking tough questions along these lines: pain doctors.

Sean Mackey, the Stanford scientist who bemoaned the lack of effective pain treatments in chapter 2, often wonders about the unconscious triggers of chronic pain. He avoids words like "nocebo," preferring more general terms like "susceptibility."

"You need to have a susceptible, vulnerable brain in place that is also taking this information and making bad things occur," he says, sitting on a patio in the hills behind the campus. "I think your brain is messing with you."

Mackey says the cutting edge of pain research is trying to understand what makes one person vulnerable and another person resilient to these deep, powerful danger signals. Of course, we can't spot those vulnerable to chronic pain any more than we can spot those prone to having placebo responses. And even if we could, they wouldn't necessarily overlap with each other, since nocebos and placebos use separate systems in the brain. But although Mackey doesn't understand what drives pain susceptibility, he's had some luck in deprogramming it and bringing relief to people who couldn't find it anywhere else.

About a decade ago, he helped create "feedback fMRI," in which patients lie in a brain scanner and attempt to control their pain by watching their own brain activity. A few years ago I visited Mackey's lab and gave the device a try for an hour or so. He started by attaching a hot metal plate to my arm to simulate the experience of chronic pain. He also spread hot pepper cream under it to further sensitize my skin. At first, it was distractingly painful. As I lay there, he told me to think of this horrible burning thing on my arm as nothing more than sunlight warmly caressing my skin. Sure enough, I watched as a part of my brain involved in pain (in that case, the anterior cingulate cortex, a couple of inches behind the left side of my forehead) slowly ramped down. Then he told me to think of it as the searing, scarring heat of a laser, and the line went up again. The way I perceived the pain instantly affected my brain's experience of it.

Mackey says this isn't proof of anything, but it does raise the question whether some chronic forms of pain originate in the brain itself. Just an old truck, stuck in a rut and unable to get out. But when he tried feedback fMRI over and over again with especially difficult chronic pain patients, he found that with practice people could alter their experience of pain by adjusting their minds—even forcing it to fade away into the background. Does this mean that chronic pain, fibromyalgia, and neuralgia are nothing but elaborate nocebos?

Is some element of chronic pain caused by negative expectation? And if so, should we be thinking more about how the brain perceives pain than about the pain itself? It's a tantalizing idea, but there's little evidence yet to confirm it. If it's true, though, then clinicians could have a powerful new approach to limiting side effects and fighting chronic pain. But with or without proof, it's still possible to use that approach to bring relief.

Christopher Spevak, a pain doctor at the Walter Reed National Military Medical Center outside Washington, D.C., has seen many patients who have suffered terrible battle wounds that have led to long-term chronic pain. Spevak can't say how much of a patient's lingering pain comes from his wound and how much comes from his mind. So he goes after both, using a traditional pharmacy as well as the patient's internal pharmacy. In a simple conditioning exercise, every time a soldier takes his traditional painkiller, it's accompanied by a particular sensory input. Perhaps it's the smell of peppermint or the taste of a strong-flavored candy or the sound of a favorite song.

The soldier begins to associate the pain relief with the flavor or the sound, and pretty soon his internal pharmacy begins to operate on the pain whenever he hears that music or tastes that flavor. And over time, that person needs less of the original drug as his mind recalibrates how it receives pain. Is Spevak reprogramming the brain to ignore a noxious nocebo? We don't know yet, but we do know that his treatment works and has improved the lives of dozens of suffering veterans.

Many cases don't even require such strong measures; sometimes the best scenario is to avoid the negative suggestion in the first place. One Harvard study looked at doctors who administered epidurals to women in labor, testing two different phrases to describe what they were doing. Simply changing their description from "a big bee sting" to "a local anesthetic that will numb the area" drastically changed how patients experienced the pain of the procedure.

There are a hundred little things doctors can do to avoid triggering a nocebo. Remember that in a doctor's office—just as in the laboratory—it takes only a few words to trigger a nocebo effect. For instance, Colloca feels that a doctor should never say "Don't worry" to a patient. Of course the patient is worried! Telling her what not to do just makes it worse. Instead, the doctor should address those fears and come up with novel ways to frame the dangers. The doctor who approaches a patient with straightforward, positive language ("Here is what is happening to you, and here is what we are going to do about it") stands a better chance of fighting off potential nocebo effects and maybe nipping chronic pain in the bud.

• • •

Nocebo effects are primeval. They originate deep in your brain and, as with placebos, happen with or without your conscious consent. We have seen how they work in the setting of a lab or a doctor's office. But their effects can be seen in the real world in almost every corner of the human experience. Nausea, immune response, and the autonomic nervous system (the part we don't consciously direct—like breathing and heartbeat) can be at the beck and call of negative expectations. But apart from pain, they can be hard to study. Can you imagine giving depressed patients a placebo and telling them it will make them more depressed? Or giving Parkinson's patients pills meant to accelerate their symptoms?

And yet, there's no question that negative expectations can play havoc with all kinds of health issues. And although it hasn't been documented, it's fair to assume that—like placebos—social pressure enhances and reinforces a nocebo. As with placebos, a good nocebo needs to tap into a powerful, plausible story with vague, placebo-prone symptoms.

For instance, in 2010 a mysterious disease of headache and abdominal pain swept through a school in rural Bangladesh after a student ate cookies from a package with a discolored label. Fears that all the cookies were somehow cursed swept across the school and then other schools in the area, sending dozens of children to the hospital. All recovered in a few hours. It wasn't the first or last time so-called mass hysteria had swept through Bangladesh. Similar events occurred in 2009, 2013, and 2016 in schools and factories around the country. Of course we can't be sure some of these people weren't genuinely sick, nor can we link the reactions directly to the kinds of nocebos we see in a laboratory. That said, among the reasons scientists say the diseases were psychosomatic are (1) like most placebos, they dissipated quickly and (2) they seemed to involve symptoms that respond to changes in expectation.

But it's not just in exotic lands that nocebo-like panics happen; they're universal. In 2007, there was a media panic in New Zealand around the idea that there was something wrong with the thyroid drug Eltroxin when the manufacturer had merely changed its color and shape. Over the course of 18 months, reports of side effects rocketed up 2,000 times.

And then there is the bizarre phenomenon of wind turbine syndrome. Led by a pediatrician named Nina Pierpont, those who insist on its existence define it as a disease caused by living near wind turbines. In the process of spinning and collecting energy, wind turbines emit a very low "infrasound," below the audible range of sound. Pierpont believes that this low-frequency hum can cause all manner of sickness, from asthma and Asperger's syndrome to anemia, allergies, and angina. And those are just the *a*'s. Pierpont has counted a whopping 223 symptoms related to inaudible turbine noises.

She published her hypothesis in a 2009 book, the media picked up on it, and the insidious disease of infrasound from wind farms spread panic like wildfire. It had all the hallmarks of a scary disease—ubiquitous, invisible, and really, really vague. It didn't matter that Pierpont doesn't have any expertise in epidemiology, acoustics, or neurology. The presence of massive spinning towers in your neighborhood can be disorienting. But then you hear about a medical condition caused by that constant whirring noise. It's invisible, incurable, and unstoppable. This powerless sense of fear births a hypervigilance in your mind. *Thrum, thrum.* I feel a cold coming on, and I have been a little tired lately. Could that be from the infrasonic vibrations? *Thrum, thrum.*

Now, there is some evidence that some people might actually be able to perceive extremely low sounds. Most men speak at around 120 hertz (which measures the frequency, or pitch, of a sound), and women at around 210 hertz. The lowest Barry White sings is about 90 hertz. Most humans can't hear anything below 20 hertz.[10]

Some researchers have observed that we can subconsciously detect sounds below this level, translating them into a vague sense of anxiety or awe, but it's not clear whether this is true. Nor is it clear that such inaudible acoustic vibrations could cause health problems at low levels, even over years. Yet thousands of people around the world are convinced that they suffer from the power of ultra-low sound waves. How can something that we may not even perceive make some of us sick and others not?

To answer this question, New Zealand researcher Keith Petrie of the University of Auckland decided to look for another cause. In 2012 he split 54 volunteers into two groups. One group was told all about the nasty dangers of wind turbines; the other was told the turbines were good for the environment. Next, both groups were exposed to ultrasonic noise on a par with that emitted by a nearby wind farm—except that half of each group just heard silence. Remember, infrasound by definition is inaudible anyway. Petrie found that people who were told the negative news about wind turbines experienced tinnitus, fatigue, concentration problems, and loss of motivation, whether they heard low-frequency noise or not. The ones who were told only positive facts about wind turbines felt less severe symptoms. But they still felt something. And that can be explained: After all, when someone asks you if you're feeling fatigued, there is a good chance you will say yes.

---

10 The world record for the lowest note produced by a human voice is less than 1 hertz, by a singer named Tim Storms. That's below the range of a human's hearing, so even he can't hear it. Elephants can communicate at around 14 hertz, but Storms's note is too low even for them.

So Petrie recruited another group of volunteers and told half of them the bad news about ultrasonic noise; he told the other half that ultrasonic noise actually eliminates health problems. Sure enough, most people responded positively to whatever suggestion they were told, regardless of what they were hearing. Petrie has replicated the experiments a couple different ways, but the results are always the same. This is not to say that the symptoms of wind turbine syndrome do not exist; indeed, many could be very real and even debilitating. It's just that they may not be caused by low-frequency noise from a nearby wind farm but rather from people's own meddlesome brains.

Infrasonic wind turbine syndrome is not alone in the modern-day world of dubious diseases. Spend just a few minutes perusing the online debates over post–Lyme disease syndrome, chronic fatigue syndrome, headaches caused by cell phone use, multiple personality disorder, or fibromyalgia and it won't be long until you find yourself neck-deep in heated controversies—not over how to treat these diseases but whether they even exist. Similar debates rage over mold allergies, trace chemicals in the environment—even electrical devices.

These sorts of conditions have varying levels of acceptance in the medical community and a wide variety of symptoms. Like wind turbine syndrome, all have mysterious mechanisms and tough pathologies to pin down. All have patients who claim that their condition has permanently altered, even crippled, them. For those of us who don't suffer from one of them, it's easy to dismiss these people as neurotic or just plain crazy. But is it possible that so many thousands of people could really be suffering under some kind of delusion? After all, just because science hasn't discovered the cause of a malady doesn't mean that the malady doesn't exist.

Or maybe we just have to redefine what *disease* means. If a disease is all in our head, does that mean it's not real? Is a psychosomatic disease that cripples a person any less debilitating than a physiological one? If you can't get out of bed, you can't get out of bed. The only difference is the way we approach treatment. We've already seen that expectation has the capacity to transform a mental state into a measurable, physiological response to ease suffering, even cure it. Those changes certainly can be permanent, and thus very real. Who's to say that it can't work the other way? And who are we to say what is real and what is fake when a soldier is suffering from intolerable pain or a woman is gasping for air on the floor of her doctor's office because of an artificial rose?

● ● ●

Our negative expectations have many forms. Take superstitions, for example; every culture has its own. Spilled salt, walking under ladders, Friday the 13th, giving a knife as a present, having a bird look directly at you—all are considered bad luck in parts of the world. In the United States, baseball pitchers argue over whether it's more unlucky to scuff the chalk baselines with their foot as they walk out to the field or purposefully not scuff it. Watch a game and you will see that almost every pitcher either scuffs or doesn't scuff. No one does both. (As a dedicated non-scuffer, I naturally distrust any pitcher who scuffs. Scuffing is the first step toward total anarchy.) And if a non-scuffer was to accidentally scuff the baseline, you can bet he wouldn't make it past the third inning. With superstition, belief and fear unite to convince a person that some supernatural influence could negatively affect something they do.

Just how strong can the power of fear be? Strong enough to kill you?

The terrifying answer: Maybe.

Walter B. Cannon was a Harvard psychologist in the first half of the 20th century who coined the phrase "fight or flight" in reference to the sympathetic nervous system—often characterized by things like adrenaline, sweat, a racing heart, and that sick taste in the back of your mouth when you are terrified. Later in his life, though, Cannon became obsessed with the notion of something he called voodoo death—namely, that a person could suffer terrible physical ailments if they believed some evil power had taken hold in them.

What are the limits of negative expectation? According to Cannon, there are none. He hypothesized that it was possible for someone to become so agitated, so frightened, that she could literally die from it. He was convinced that if that happened, it would appear in the black magic of various "aborigines," by which he seems to have meant pretty much any impoverished, poorly educated community that uses folk healing. In 1942 he argued that under the right circumstances, a well-placed curse or bit of bad luck could so frighten a person within a specific cultural context that her system would literally shut down from stress.

It was a fascinating idea, and for decades anthropologists and psychologists argued about whether it was possible. Some said extreme stress or hopelessness or fear, coupled with not eating, could drive a person to die in a matter of days. Others said this was just a fantasy cooked up by wealthy countries to make their poorer counterparts seem exotic. Yet, tragic events caused by the power of negativity aren't limited to one culture. In the Western world we see a tendency for elderly spouses to die in quick succession—the second said to die from a broken heart. People who consider themselves at risk for heart disease die four times more often than similarly healthy people who don't think they're at risk. And certainly people with cancer who have a dim outlook on their future don't live as long as optimistic patients. In Cambodia, during the horrendous 1975–79 reign of the Khmer Rouge, women who had watched their husbands and children butchered before their eyes reportedly became blind; it was said they wept until they could no longer see.

But killing an otherwise healthy young person with just suggestion? That's something else. In her fascinating book *Sleep Paralysis: Night-Mares, Nocebos, and the Mind-Body Connection,* Shelley Adler identifies a modern-day sort of voodoo death among Laotian immigrants to the United States. She writes about members of the Hmong communities who died from their belief that ghosts were haunting them just as they woke up. She chalks up the phenomenon to a deep-seated fear resulting in a very real condition in which people are momentarily unable to move either just as they fall asleep or just as they wake up. Such paralysis, often accompanied by ethereal hallucinations, can be traumatic for anyone (and may be the root of many alien abduction stories). It's not clear how people die from sleep-paralysis terror or why so many of them hail from the hill communities of Laos. But in the right cultural context, it's conceivable that fear can kill a person.

Christian Scientists have their own version of this belief. In an oft-quoted story about the lethal power of negative expectation, the religion's founder, Mary Baker Eddy, wrote of a man who was told that he had slept in a bed where another man had just died of cholera. He quickly came down with symptoms of cholera and died a couple of hours later—before it came to light that no such person had ever slept on that bed. Now, it's not clear if this ever really happened. And it's highly unlikely that you could catch cholera from sleeping in an infected person's bed (cholera is found in feces and is generally transmitted through contaminated water, not from fleas or bedbugs). Plus, a couple of hours is pretty fast for someone to catch and die from cholera. It is indeed a dangerous disease but isn't lethal on its own; what kills people is usually dehydration from the prolific diarrhea resulting from it.

The point is that during the 19th century, cholera was a terrifying and mysterious disease—and that the fear of it alone might have been suggestion enough to kill someone. This, I was told, was the kind of thing that could happen when a Christian Scientist let down his guard: Suggestion could literally kill you. And for a little kid growing up in a religious world dominated by the invisible power of the mind, this idea was terrifying.

But it wasn't just the vague, societal fear of disease that could get me; there was also a more targeted kind. "Mental malpractice," as it was called, was the act of wishing someone ill and thus causing him to get ill, or worse. In other words, a Christian Science version of a curse. To fight mental malpractice, my mom always quoted the church's founder, saying I had to "stand porter at the door of thought." This means blocking all aggressive thoughts, either free-floating or targeted by someone who wished me ill. I didn't fully understand it at the time, but it made a pretty powerful impression on a little kid. Whenever I got sick, I spent a fair amount of time imagining British Queen's Guards standing inside my ears, just in case.

These ideas are not unique to Christian Scientists. In many cultures, tragic events are broken into two loose groups: generalized evil from which you must regularly protect yourself, and targeted evil from sinister supernatural or human actors. Expectation certainly plays a role in the former, but what about the latter? Here, the already thin trickle of scholarship on negative expectation runs dry. Getting sick from fear is not the same as getting sick from the ill will of another person. For that, we have to move into uncharted territory.

Almost every culture on earth has its own language of curses. Hexes, bad juju, demons, djinn, black magic—when you get sick, it has never been hard to find someone to blame. To be clear, a curse is not a nocebo. But if you believe you've been cursed, the nocebo effect certainly plays a role in any resulting changes to your health. Curses are unique to each culture, but they often involve a powerful source of evil and a victim who is not adequately protected from harm. In my community growing up, people wouldn't actually accuse one another of mental malpractice—after all, this was suburban California in the 1980s, not Salem, Massachusetts, in the 1690s. But it was occasionally whispered about when someone suddenly became sick.

Among the many curses of the occult world, the most famous—the one that spawned an entire genre of movies, books, and TV shows—is the zombie curse of Haiti. According to legend, those people who find themselves on the wrong side of a Haitian medicine man, or *bokor*, will die from his curse. These people will be buried in a grave and after a set period will be uncovered by the *bokor*, neither dead nor living, and forced to work as a slave to the *bokor*. Although this is a staple of the Hollywood entertainment machine, there have been only a handful of documented cases of zombies, going back to 1937. In all these cases, the subjects shared the same general symptoms: the inability to speak more than a few words, cognitive impairments, and walking with a pronounced shuffle. In 1997 the medical journal *The Lancet* even published descriptions of three cases of zombies (two of which seemed to mistake the identity of those mental disabilities).

Now, there are two complementary theories as to how one might go about creating a zombie. The first is that *bokors use puffer fish venom to* simulate death. Then the lack of oxygen from the time spent buried in a wooden boxed causes brain damage and that telltale shuffle. The second explanation is much more fascinating. Some have suggested that the tremendous cultural pressure to become a zombie after being knocked out and buried might have actually forced the poor wretch to turn himself into a shuffling creature of scorn. In other words, zombies could be self-made, molded from the collective will of a community—a massive, societal negative expectation fulfilled.

Of course, this is all conjecture. In the laboratory, we know that nocebos can be initiated with just a few well-placed words. And we know that societal pressures can heighten placebos. But what do we know about the history of curses thousands of years old? To get a little clarity on the power of negative expectation on the human body, I call up one of the masters of placebo and nocebo research, Jon-Kar Zubieta, a professor at the University of Michigan.

Zubieta has done pioneering work inducing nocebos to infer their mechanisms and differentiate them from placebos. He's an expert in the power of the mind to affect the body. We talk for a while about his work in the lab with Parkinson's patients and pain, and then the conversation turns to black magic.

"Let's say, for example, you go to a faith healer, and the faith healer tells you, 'This is going to be great, and this works fantastically, and you will feel better, and everything's good,' " Zubieta says to me. "But you could go to someone who says, 'And by the way, you are a bad person, and you are cursed.' And if you believe it, you are screwed." He pauses. "But I think to do that experimentally is a little bit difficult."

I laugh at the image of a bunch of people in lab coats surrounding a witch doctor, burning candles, and hexing a person in the next room. And then I get a wonderful, terrible idea. I may not have a laboratory setting, and I may not be a scientist, but I have two things those people don't: access to practitioners of the occult and an extremely bad sense of judgment. I decide to hire someone to put a curse on me.

I don't believe in curses per se, but like any good scientist, I don't know what I don't know. I'm pretty sure that no matter what I believe a curse over my head will weigh on my mind. If I'm lucky, I'll be able to experience the hypervigilance that comes from negative expectations. If I'm even luckier, maybe I'll feel the unconscious effect of a nocebo. And if I'm really lucky, maybe I'll even get sick or develop some mysterious type of chronic pain.

This is the special type of idiot that I am.

Living in Mexico City, I'm a short train ride away from scores of brujos. For the right price, any one of them will happily put a curse on my head. I float the idea by a few friends, who act as if I'm planning to go to Syria to interview terrorists. In an online chat, I mention it to a journalist—a photographer and a veteran of multiple war zones.

"You're about to have a baby," he writes. I tell him that my wife won't be coming (but I don't share that she's dead set against it). There's a long pause and then: "This could be the worst idea you've ever had. What if you die? I mean, look at the Kennedys."

It's true that an oddly high number of Kennedy family members did seem to meet an early end, but I hardly subscribe to the popular notion of a "Kennedy curse." An online search turns up a flood of fringe conspiracy theories, seemingly spun around two potential causes of the Kennedys' bad luck. One is that the family patriarch, Joe Kennedy, was once rude to a Holocaust survivor and thus brought decades of death and destruction to his family. The other is that an earlier member of the Kennedy clan accidentally stepped on the home of a family of fairies back in Ireland. Fairies, it seems, know how to hold a grudge.

The Kennedy family's bad luck is actually a telling example of the true nature of curses. You see, curses aren't magical; they're statistical. They rely on the fact that—as should be evident by this point—we are not always rational creatures. If we were all equipped with perfectly logical minds, we would see that the number of bad things happening to people who've been cursed is the same as the number of bad things happening to everyone else.

But that's not how our minds work. More often, we look for bad things and then work backward. It's a very old logical fallacy. The Romans called it *post hoc, ergo propter hoc*, meaning "after this, therefore because of this." If a piano falls on your head, it's because you walked under a ladder two weeks ago. Never mind that many people who work in the ladder industry, regularly use ladders, or just happen to walk under them every day manage to avoid falling pianos.

But the idea of some origin curse leading to a family's misfortune is emotionally powerful. And like nocebos, it's an idea that relies on fear rather than hope. Ask yourself this: If someone tells you you're blessed, would that hit you with the same emotional power as someone telling you you're cursed? This is the theme that seems to follow all kinds of negative expectations, be they curses, mass hysteria, or laboratory nocebos: They have an immediacy that positive expectations just don't.

Perhaps it's my Christian Science childhood whispering in my ear to "stand porter"; perhaps it's just overconfidence. But after being universally told it's a bad idea, I decide to go to get myself cursed.

• • •

From the front, Mercado Sonora looks like any other bustling market in Mexico City. Concrete building, fluorescent lighting, row after row of piñatas, cheap designer knock-off jeans, and poofy quinceañera dresses on so many mannequins that it looks like an army of decapitated Disney princesses. But walk back far enough, past the industrial bags of birdseed, live chickens and rabbits, and dried chilies, and you get to the brujo market.

Here, instead of tiaras and Spider-Man piñatas, you'll find dried snakeskins and coyote heads; in place of cheap plastic toys, ghoulish blackened dolls used for summoning evil spirits. You can buy ointments in every stall, receive blessings, and occasionally destroy your enemies. In short, this is the place for all your magical needs.

Standing outside the market, I'm surprisingly nervous, but curiosity and pride force me ahead. The first task is to check in with the communications office. That's right: Mexico City's largest witchcraft market has a public relations arm. My translator and I go to the drab office and meet bureaucrats who seem mildly interested in what we are doing and then ask us to sign in. *Curses? Yes, yes, very scary. Go ahead and sign here. Will you be using video cameras? Good, just fill out this form.*

Paperwork complete, we ask around and easily find our way to Manuel Valadez, a second-generation brujo with a broad smile. He welcomes us to his tiny store and begins telling of his craft. He was not born to the calling, he says, but learned witchcraft by studying under his aunt. He's an affable man with a button-down shirt, a bronze dragon bracelet, and a necklace of tiny carved skulls. He's portly and cheerful and seems more like a grandfatherly hippie than he does a master of the occult. He invites us to the back of his small shop, which is sprinkled with candles, oils, and statues of Santa Muerte, the saint of death. (Santa Muerte is not recognized by the pope but is enormously popular in Mexico and looks a little like the Grim Reaper.)

"The world has both good and evil," Valadez says. "To build something, you must first destroy."

Valadez says that the ingredients of his treatments are important but not the most crucial part of his work. "Nothing in this works if you don't have faith. Faith is like the engine," he tells me.

I realize this last part might be a problem for me but decide to overlook it for now. Finally I muster the courage to ask Valadez if he'll agree to curse *me*. He is silent for a long moment.

"You mean, you want to be like a guinea pig?" he asks, perplexed. "I like you. I don't want to curse you. Why invite aggression?"

I convince him, promising to have him lift the curse after a few days.

The administration of a curse is a surprisingly simple thing. I don't even have to be in the room. Valadez has me write my name on a little white strip, he burns it in a special black candle, and he calls upon the spirits to cause problems in my life. That's it. Across Latin America, this theme of a paper with your name on it is common. Some believe if you freeze a paper with a person's name on it, they will be cursed until you thaw it out. (When the Americans finally caught up with drug trafficker and Panamanian dictator Manuel Noriega, it's said that his freezer was full of pieces of paper with names, encased in ice cubes.)

I go home feeling exactly the same as when I'd arrived. In fact, for most of the week, I forget that I've been cursed. I do wake up the day after the encounter with a splitting headache (though that might have been from the bottle of single malt Scotch I helped consume the night before at a friend's birthday party). Then, out of the blue, my electric toothbrush stops working, even though I just recharged it. Later I have a coughing fit that leads to hiccups for a minute. And a few days afterward, I go to the dentist and find out I might need a root canal (though, if I'm honest, this wasn't really a huge surprise).

As the week goes on, I grow more and more confident. I think about the curse once while riding my bike down a busy street at night, but I shake it off and just keep a sharp eye on cross traffic. When I return to Valadez's stall the following Friday, I'm ready to call the whole thing a bust.

But Valadez isn't there. His assistant says that he'll be dealing with a family emergency until Tuesday. I shrug and figure another weekend of lingering curse can't hurt me any more than the previous week has.

As if to tempt fate, that Saturday I enjoy a day of rock climbing in a forested canyon just outside town. Though it's rainy season, and I am recuperating from an ankle injury, the day is uneventful and pleasant. But that night, my wife, now four months pregnant, feels a persistent pain in her abdomen. Sunday morning, we call the doctor, who prescribes an over-the-counter muscle relaxant and tells us to call her if the pain doesn't go away. By one o'clock, it hasn't eased, and the doctor tells us to go to the emergency room. She's worried that the pain—whatever initiated it—could be transforming into contractions.

Riding in a taxi across our neighborhood to the emergency room, I try to console my distraught wife. But in the back of my mind, as if patiently sitting on a chair in the corner of my subconscious, one thought presents itself: What if this is the curse? What kind of horrible hubris has led me to this point?

In that moment I truly understand the power of nocebos—of that old Roman phrase *post hoc, ergo propter hoc.* If something happens to my child, regardless of the cause, my wife will never forgive me. I will certainly never forgive myself. The curse is no more powerful in that moment than it has been the previous week. It hasn't caused me to slip and bump my head or weakened my immune system. And it certainly doesn't have the power to harm my child. No, the real power of a curse is to give cause to a bad event—to give me someone to blame. In this case, myself.

That's how quickly a man of science can turn to superstition.

Whether it's a curse or a blessing, the power of belief comes from two little words: *What if?* What if that blessing could have helped me get the job I wanted? What if that ex-girlfriend I cheated on five years ago decided to curse me? What if my great-great-grandfather accidentally killed a bunch of fairies? What if black cats really are bad luck? What if my unborn child dies and it is my fault?

We get to the hospital and face the usual barrage of red tape. But when a doctor sees my pregnant wife weeping, she whisks her away while I fill out paperwork. For a few nightmarish minutes, the obstetrician on call can't find the baby's heartbeat. Seconds tick by and the doctor gets increasingly frustrated until she finally finds it.

It turns out the pain wasn't in the uterus but in the stomach—a result of stretching ligaments mixed with a plate of tacos from the day before that aren't sitting well. The baby is healthy. The doctors take us up to the sonogram room, and I watch as they inspect my child and confirm that everything is just fine.

They tell us the baby is a boy. And as I sit there in the darkened room, staring at an image of my son stretching his arms, all thought of supernatural evil power disappears. The doctors and I joke in Spanish as they try to get a 3-D snapshot of my squirming son's face. He is perfect, healthy, and exactly as he should be.

On that Sunday in June—my first Father's Day—I feel anything but cursed.

● ● ●

A few days later I return to Valadez's stall and ask him to lift the curse. He says a few prayers, lights a cigar, blows the smoke over me, and gives me a candle that needs to be lit on top of some money and a photo of myself. He asks me how my week went—if I had any bad luck. I tell him yes, but don't mention our scare. I certainly don't blame the curse for our trip to the hospital, but I figure he might. And I'm not sure how he would feel about the idea of his magic endangering an unborn baby.

In the end, the only difference between a curse and a blessing was what I brought to it. It reminded me of some of the many studies with placebos and pain. In a split second, pain can switch from placebo to nocebo with just a suggestion. It reminded me of being inside Sean Mackey's real-time fMRI machine, where a simple change in how I thought about that heated pad on my arm changed the sensation from feeling warm sun to laser-like pain.

We are programmed to fear first and have hope later, as long as we're sure there's nothing to fear. As a rock climber and now a journalist, I have spent my adult life fighting against fear in hopes of finding a higher, more profound reward. But in my deepest subconscious—where nocebos and self-doubt run free—I am as much a slave to fear as anyone.

We are who we are, no matter how that might conflict with who we think we are. Our suggestibility to manipulations, whether positive or negative, is fundamental to being human. And what looks like magic is often just our own frightened, malleable brains casting about for a way to explain what's going on around us. We are, all of us, storytellers, and the most powerful story we have is the one we tell ourselves.

But one type of story is even more powerful at harnessing our expectation than either placebos or nocebos. So powerful that with just a few spoken words, it can erase pain, memories, and even disfiguring skin diseases.

So powerful, in fact, it's hard to argue that it's not magic.

CHAPTER FIVE

You *Are* Getting Sleepy . . .

*Everything that has been said and written
about the great dangers of hypnosis belongs
to the realm of fable.*

—Sigmund Freud

L ONG BEFORE WE KNEW ANYTHING about placebos, dopamine, or fMRI machines, scientists had one singularly powerful tool to understand suggestibility and expectation. Those wanting to explore the mind's connection to the body had to enter the dark and sordid world of hypnosis. It's hard to imagine anything more closely tied to suggestibility than hypnotic susceptibility. Hypnosis has inspired scientists and snake oil salesmen alike for centuries, and it holds fascinating clues into the world of suggestion and expectation in the brain. It's a powerful, tangible phenomenon that has cured addiction, erased pain, and brought comfort to millions. And while it's easy enough to perform on a Las Vegas stage, we still don't really understand how it works.

More than one scientist has attempted to link hypnosis and placebos; both seem especially effective against pain, anxiety, and sleep problems. Both utilize complex brain processes based on expectation that are not fully understood. Throughout history, both of them have been stigmatized and co-opted into superstition and magic. Hypnotizable people, as with people who are placebo prone, are often seen by mainstream culture as somewhat weak-minded. And just as with placebos, nothing could be further from the truth.

With both hypnosis and the placebo effect, people rely on nothing but their own brains, mixed with a little suggestion, to yield sometimes dramatic results. And for a long time, both were considered fringe. But in the past few years, placebos have come closer to mainstream acceptance, whereas hypnosis is still rarely taken seriously. This is in part because of the checkered history of hypnosis and in part because, unlike the placebo effect, hypnosis has stubbornly refused to reveal its mechanism. However, in recent decades scientists have been able to glean a few tidbits that suggest a potential a brain-based understanding of the ancient practice.

Experts who study what happens during hypnosis fall into two loose camps. One group asserts that hypnosis is a form of intense focus, like daydreaming or getting lost in a good book or jigsaw puzzle. For many people, that's all hypnosis is: a nice relaxing meditation, a little like the end of a yoga session, when everybody gets to lie down and focus on breathing. For them, hypnosis is like lying in the grass on a sunny spring day, staring into a cloud so intently that you momentarily lose yourself in it. It's not a state unfamiliar to real life. For others, hypnosis can be much, much more. The second group of scientists considers it an "altered state," having no counterpart in daily life. Some people under hypnosis commune with the dead, revisit their past, and perform superhuman feats. Warts disappear from their skin, and they feel no pain when surgeons slice into them.

How can one person feel nothing but pleasant relaxation while another can hallucinate or be rendered mute just from listening to someone speak? All we can say with any confidence is that hypnosis is a form of focus—usually directed by someone describing a soothing narrative—that causes some people to enter a trance-like state in which their minds are open to outside suggestion. One thing that is certain is that, just as with placebos, the element of storytelling is crucial to hypnosis. In the case of placebos, that means painting a worldview of how a certain remedy could help you: Ginseng taps into your chi; homeopathic treatment cancels out the childhood fears that haunt you. Hypnosis, on the other hand, presents an actual story, painting pictures of magical places that relax you and prepare you for suggestion: walking through a field of flowers or descending a staircase or floating through space and becoming relaxed.

Of course, anyone can tell you to close your eyes and imagine walking down a staircase or floating in the clouds. But the ability to tell an evocative story—one that captures your imagination and draws you in completely—is what marks a good hypnotist. You need to get so drawn in by the voice and the images that you lose yourself for a moment and become more suggestible. You're still conscious, just listening differently. What is suggestion but the stories we tell ourselves mixed with the stories others are telling us?

● ● ●

There is no consensus on who first practiced the art of hypnosis. The novelist and poet Sir Walter Scott referenced it in 1805, noting that Gypsies among certain rural Scottish communities had "the power of throwing upon bystanders a spell to fascinate their eyes and cause them to see the thing that is not." But neither he, nor anyone of his time, knew where it had come from. Some scholars have hypothesized that the practice goes back to ancient Egypt or Greece. But the more likely scenario is that the Roma (or Gypsies, as they are often incorrectly called) brought it to Europe from their original home in India a thousand years ago. Whatever its roots, hypnosis became entrenched in the cultural consciousness as both a medical treatment and a cool parlor trick.

About 30 years before Scott, our old friend Franz Mesmer practiced hypnotism, though under another name. As you'll recall, Mesmer's "animal magnetism" wasn't just about using mental powers to magnetize water; it was also about magnetizing people directly. Using nothing but his captivating voice, Mesmer could in a matter of minutes cause people to fall into trances, have convulsions, even lose their power of speech.

Mesmer claimed that the effect—what later became known as mesmerism—was the result of the overpowering control of the magnet juice he aimed at his patients. The truth is that he had stumbled on a very real neurological phenomenon, which fell out of favor when he did. But mesmerism resurfaced in the mid-1800s when an English surgeon named James Braid coined the term "hypnosis." He rejected both the magnet idea and the notion that its power came from the hypnotist. Braid flipped that notion around and said that the trance had more to do with the person being hypnotized.

More impressively, Braid and other scientists became expert hypnotists, even using hypnosis for surgery.[11] Anesthesiology didn't yet exist—an anesthesiologist was the guy who brought you a bottle of whiskey and told you to bite down on a stick. But with hypnosis, it was possible to pull teeth—or, in one case, amputate a leg—painlessly while a patient was in a trance. For the next few decades, hypnosis became so widespread that even Sigmund Freud studied it. Nobel laureate Charles Richet, a contemporary of Freud's and one of the most prominent psychologists of the day, was also a prominent hypnotist.

---

11 Well into the 20th century, hypnosis was used in childbirth, especially in Russia. Stalin himself was a quite a fan.

But although hypnotists were becoming more respected in the late 1880s, people who were easily hypnotized were not. A physician writing in *The American Naturalist* in 1882 put it this way: "In the mesmerism of men, those whose minds are naturally weak, or who have become enfeebled by disease, are the ones most easily controlled."

For whatever reason, soon after the turn of the 20th century, hypnosis began its slow, steady nosedive in public opinion, thanks in part to its long-standing association with charlatans and con men. The greatest of these was Walford Bodie, an uncanny hypnotist, performer, medical fraud, and womanizer who became celebrated for his hypnosis performances in the late 1800s. An inspiration to both Harry Houdini and Charlie Chaplin, Bodie would use hypnosis to "heal" people on stage or perform bloodless surgeries. Most of this was a complete sham—Bodie liberally mixed hypnosis with stage tricks. Some of his hypnosis was certainly real, but an astute viewer might have noticed that the same "volunteer" would get mesmerized to walk like a chicken night after night.

At the same time that Bodie was turning hypnosis into entertainment, many scientists were eager to study the phenomenon. Baron Albert von Schrenck-Notzing, (nicknamed Baron "Shrinks at Nothing"), a notable German gentleman scientist who studied alongside Freud, spent decades with various magicians and fortune-tellers, one of whom supposedly released bizarre smoky plasma from her bodily orifices while hypnotized. Pretty soon, researchers began expanding this sort of research to ghosts, magic, and monsters as well. Trances led to séances and then demonic possession. Some of the enthusiasm came from so much new technology—the sense that with the recent advent of human flight, electricity, and vaccines, anything was possible. But some of it came from not having the right technology to investigate the human mind properly. These investigators witnessed many incredible demonstrations of hypnotism's power but in the end were no closer to understanding how the phenomenon works than their counterparts had been a hundred years earlier.

Oddly enough, Christian Science shares a link with these early days of hypnosis. Its founder, Mary Baker Eddy, was introduced to faith healing through a hypnotist named Phineas Quimby. In addition to having one of the top 10 greatest names in history, Quimby was the student of a student of Mesmer's and had helped Eddy with numerous ailments she had suffered since childhood. For a while, Eddy seemed taken with the man's abilities to bring comfort to his patients. But as Christian Science became more popular and independent in its own right, she made a public break with her mentor's methods, even codifying her antipathy for hypnotism as the subject of one of her weekly Bible lessons that Christian Scientists read to this day.

Eddy wasn't alone. Most orthodox Christians and Muslims eventually rejected and continue to reject hypnosis as a tool of Satan or supernatural creatures called djinn. (One hypnotist, who works in a hospital easing people's pain, told me he commonly meets patients who refuse his help on religious grounds. A few have even made the sign of the cross to ward him off, as if he were a vampire.) Mainstream science and popular culture shared this view, thanks in part to widely publicized stories of the lethal power of hypnosis. In 1894, a 22-year-old Hungarian noblewoman died in a séance, supposedly from its effects. The following year, George du Maurier published a wildly popular serial, *Trilby*, in which a hypnotist named Svengali seduces and manipulates an impressionable young Englishwoman through hypnosis. Thus began a long history of evil hypnotists in pop culture who influence their victims to rob banks, kill people, and (naturally) fall in love with the hypnotist.

By the time moving pictures were born, an archetype had been built. *Trilby* has been adapted for the screen at least eight times, while many TV series (among them *Gilligan's Island, Colombo,* and *Scooby-Doo*) have propagated the "evil hypnotist" trope. Interestingly, in Bram Stoker's 1897 novel *Dracula,* it was the hero who used hypnosis to find the vampire. But by the time the various movie versions came along, it was always the bloodsucker himself who hypnotized his victims. In the 2013 movie *Now You See Me,* a stage magician hypnotizes a guy on the street into robbing his own bank. In *The Manchurian Candidate,* a man is programmed to kill the president. The classic Hollywood hypnotist has a goatee and swirling spirals in his eyes, and may (as in the 1999 movie *Office Space*) inadvertently leave a victim permanently changed or damaged. For much of the 20th century, it was actually illegal in Britain to show hypnosis on television for fear that someone might entrance viewers against their will.[12]

Although highly entertaining, the Hollywood version of hypnosis proved to be far from accurate (much as it is for amnesia, voodoo, and attractive women falling for Adam Sandler). Any hypnosis researcher can tell you that hypnotists don't wield omnipotent power, as they do in the movies. You can't hypnotize people against their will. You can't make people do something they wouldn't want to do. You can't turn someone into your personal slave.

But over the years, hypnosis has never shaken its dubious history, and so remains on the fringes of science and society. Every few decades it seems there is a resurgence of interest in the subject—and whenever that happens, scientists glimpse a phenomenon with extraordinary power over the body. A few of these stories simply defy belief.

● ● ●

---

12 The Hypnotism Act of 1952 was designed to "regulate the demonstration of hypnotic phenomena for purposes of public entertainment." The act required a special permit to allow hypnotists to practice in public but was vague about what was allowed and what was not, since its creators obviously had no idea what hypnotism was. It has been ratified several times since but is still completely bizarre and lives in a legal gray area.

In 1951, England was still recovering from the devastation of World War II. Young boys had to make toys from used munitions and playgrounds from the rotting hulks of buildings that still littered parts of the country. It was a hard place to grow up, and perhaps none had it harder than 16-year-old F. T. Moore, who suffered from a rare congenital case of ichthyosiform erythroderma, which roughly translates to "fishlike skin." The condition starts out as slightly tough skin that's a little darker than normal. From there, it expands into lesions that the *British Medical Journal* describes as a "black, horny layer covering the entire body except for the chest, neck and face." Moore's lesions were hard, like fingernails, and especially thick on the boy's feet, palms, and thighs; they constantly cracked and became infected, oozing a "bloodstained serum" whose odor nauseated not only Moore but his classmates as well. The parts that were not cracked and painful were completely numb. Because of his shocking appearance, pungent smell, and near constant pain, Moore had to be pulled out of school at a young age.

Some of the top plastic surgeons at the time attempted skin grafts from parts of the boy's body that were not affected by the lesions. But every time they moved skin from a healthy part of the body to a diseased portion, the healthy skin became covered in the dark, horny lesions as well. When the surgeons gave up, Moore was taken to a physician and hypnotist named Albert A. Mason, who saw this as a unique opportunity to document the power of hypnosis on skin conditions. So Mason treated just the boy's left arm, hypnotizing Moore and planting the suggestion in the boy's mind that his arm should clear itself of the painful growths.

After the boy had endured 16 years of misery, in less than a week the scales on his arm loosened and peeled off, exposing soft, almost totally healthy skin beneath. The hypnotist next treated his right arm, then his legs, then the trunk of his body. After each treatment, broad swaths of the young man's scaly dermis came sloughing off. His legs, which had been completely covered, dropped 50 to 70 percent of their lesions. His back, which had been only lightly covered, lost 90 percent. And his arms and hands, once covered in scaly growths, lost 95 to 100 percent of their lesions. Rarely does a scientific paper bring tears to your eyes, but it's hard not to get a little misty when reading the August 23, 1952, issue of the *British Medical Journal.* Mason noted that this poor kid, who was once "lonely, solitary, with a hopeless attitude towards future friendship and employment," suddenly became a "happy, normal boy" who went on to become an electrician's assistant and then a bike mechanic with no sign of relapse.

Had it been a priest performing the hypnosis and not a doctor, it would be enough to make a person believe in God (or devise some wild explanation involving magnets). But amazing as this account is, it hasn't inspired the kind of research it deserves. Over the next half century, medical science came only marginally closer to understanding the potential power of hypnosis to heal.

A few curious researchers, however, did take up these questions. In the late 1950s and early 1960s several teams at Stanford and Harvard came up with 12-step scales to quantify how suggestible to hypnosis a person is. They devised a series of tasks to be performed under hypnosis that would reveal one's level of suggestibility. For example, in the fourth step, a hypnotist would try to immobilize your arm; in the ninth, attempt to create the hallucination that you were flying; and in the twelfth, try to cause temporary amnesia. People who rated lower on the scale might feel their arm lift on its own at the hypnotist's suggestion, while those who rated higher might lose their power of speech. Over time, it emerged that hypnotizability, or "hypnotic susceptibility," as scientists call it, seems to be a fixed trait. Ernest Hilgard at Stanford established that, as with IQ, people's susceptibility to hypnosis doesn't change much from late adolescence until the day they die. Contrary to Hollywood portrayals, the most spectacular forms of hypnosis work only on the most hypnotizable 10 percent or so of the population. Another 10 percent don't respond to hypnosis at all, and the rest fall somewhere in between.

We've also gleaned other useful information. In 1997, Canadian psychologist Pierre Rainville successfully hypnotized one group not to feel any pain from hot water poured on their hands and another group to believe they could feel the pain but that it wouldn't bother them. Then he scanned their brains with positron emission tomography and saw two very different neural reactions to pain, suggesting that the sensation of pain and the emotions associated with it have separate triggers. It also showed just how crucial emotion is to our experience of pain.

Thanks to work like Rainville's, we now know that hypnosis often involves parts of the brain associated with attention, emotion regulation, and pain. We know that people seem to be wired differently for hypnosis, and that this doesn't tend to change much over their lives. We also know your capacity to be hypnotized isn't tied to your intelligence, willpower, likelihood of crying at weddings, or tendency to listen to boy bands.

This, for many scientists, has been the most frustrating part of understanding hypnosis: recognizing and separating who is most suggestible. It's the same story we observed with placebo responders, with about the same level of success. Try as they might, scientists can't seem to identify any mental or physical trait that links reliably to hypnotizability. Some have noticed that hypnotizable people are easily distracted or "dreamy." Or that they tend to be able to focus easily. Others say they were the kind of child who had imaginary friends. A 1930 study suggested a link to extroversion and how much your body sways while you stand still. Another controversial theory from the 1970s ties hypnotizability to how much white is visible around your iris when you roll your eyes up. (The notion that a mental process could be reflected in an external feature is a little too much like phrenology for my tastes. But still . . . what if?)

One commonly used survey called the Tellegen Absorption Scale (invented in 1974 by the brilliant, and oddly named, Auke Tellegen at the University of Minnesota) attempts to bring together every factor that seems to influence hypnosis. It asks, for example, whether you are the kind of person who stares for long periods of time at clouds in the sky or at crackling fires. Do you get totally absorbed in music and sunsets? Have you ever become lost in a character you played onstage? Have you ever had an out-of-body experience or felt the presence of "someone who is not physically there"? Answering yes to some of these questions presumably indicates you have a high hypnotic susceptibility.

So if hypnosis is a brain-based phenomenon capable of healing in certain cases, and some people experience it more strongly than others, isn't it just another placebo? There are no easy answers, but the consensus today seems to be that the two are not related. For one thing, hypnotic susceptibility remains relatively stable throughout one's life, whereas placebo responsiveness can change from day to day. Also, the drug naloxone, which is effective at blocking placebo responses, doesn't block hypnosis. So if hypnosis isn't a placebo, just what is it?

To find some answers, I sit down with retired Harvard psychologist Irving Kirsch at his favorite Turkish restaurant on the outskirts of Boston. Kirsch studied placebos decades before it was fashionable for scientists to do so and is one of the country's leading experts on hypnosis. He's largely retired and has scaled back his publishing,[13] but he's as sharp as a whip and his understanding of placebos is encyclopedic. In addition to being a pioneer in placebo research, he is a

---

13 Most of this focuses on his deep antipathy for the way depression drugs are used in this country. Depression is highly suggestible, and as we've seen, drugs like Prozac don't perform terribly well against placebos. For a guy who spent his life studying sugar pills, he knows one when he sees one.

talented hypnotist who for years has searched for a link between hypnosis and placebos.

I try to explain my attempts to understand what hypnosis is doing in the brain.

"Can I try something?" he asks. "Here, put your leg on the floor and put your hand on your knee, just like that."

I realize with a thrill he's about to hypnotize me on the spot. As instructed, I plant my foot on the floor. He tells me to imagine that my foot is glued to the floor. Stuck. A lead weight. Then he asks me to try to lift it. As much as I would like to believe I am hypnotized, I lift it without a problem. Next, he asks me to put my hand on my knee and push down hard, then try to lift it. As expected, it's difficult to lift and I struggle against my hand. He tells me to memorize that feeling, internalize it.

Because it's not real. Try it yourself: Push down on your knee. Your arm isn't nearly strong enough at that angle to stop you from lifting your leg, no matter how hard you push—unless your focus is on your arm and your expectation is that it will be. Kirsch has tricked me into thinking my arm is stronger than it is by tinkering with my expectations. In a way, he says, that's what hypnosis is.

Kirsch admits that placebos and hypnosis are not the same. But they both tap into a deep force in the brain: expectation. "When you are doing something that affects people's expectations, you are changing things in the brain in a way that's related to fundamental function of the brain," he tells me. "That may in fact make placebo effects paradigmatic of how the brain produces experiences."

Remember, the brain is an expectation-prediction machine. Kirsch observes that hypnosis, like placebos, messes with the very purpose of your brain. Thus, while they are certainly separate phenomena, their differences probably aren't as important as their similarities—which in turn gives us a glimpse of the very fundamentals of consciousness.

At the end of the meal, over tea, Kirsch summarizes by paraphrasing a colleague, psychologist Marcel Kinsbourne.

"There is a wave of bottom-up information coming up from the external world, up into your brain," he tells me. "There is a wave of information coming from the cortex that consists of your evaluations, your beliefs, your expectations. Consciousness is these two waves hitting each other. It's a collision."

That, he says, is where hypnosis and placebos do their work.

● ● ●

But, of course, Kirsch's style of hypnosis is not the only kind. History has demonstrated both clinical hypnosis and, well, performance hypnosis. Nothing has both enhanced and destroyed the reputation of hypnosis as much as its practice in a performance setting. Believe it or not, the stage hypnotist can tell us a lot about our suggestible brains. So I turn to a master—someone whose livelihood depends on the ability to quickly and reliably put someone in a trance.

The British stage hypnotist Andrew Newton claims on his website to have hypnotized more than 60,000 people over the course of his 35-year career. He has performed across the world—in lonely dive bars, at packed concert halls, on television, and everything in between. Everything Newton does, wears, and says before a show is meant to build expectation in the mind of the viewer. For instance, for a time he drove a Rolls-Royce just so he could park it right in front of the theater.

"Everybody going into that theater looks at that Rolls-Royce and thinks, 'Whoa, he must be good.' This is all part of the show. The show starts when they are queuing outside to get in," he says.

And if the venue isn't full, Newton figures out a way to fill it, even giving away tickets. This not only makes the audience think the man on stage is a serious professional, it also creates a sense of community within the building, a belief in the hive mind of the viewers that the hypnotist has total power. Before each performance, Newton comes onstage to get the crowd warmed up. Different performers have different tricks, but the key is to get the audience to act as one: Get them to stand up and then sit down on your command. Get them to laugh together.

Newton, a keen observer of human behavior, says this works because humans evolved in communities. We can't help it; we want to be a part of the crowd. By signaling to the audience that he is their leader, Newton primes them to obey his suggestions. When it's really working, he says, the hypnotist is even more amazed than the audience.

Newton begins by asking for a group of volunteers. Most stage hypnotists won't risk using a single volunteer—he or she might panic, play dead, not want to cooperate, or be among the 10 percent of people who are not hypnotizable. As the group comes up to the stage, he watches them closely. It's crucial that his first act goes off perfectly to maintain the suggestion that he is in control of the hall. He says he looks for a group of kids snickering to themselves as they walk up the stairs. If they get to the stage and blanch a little at the hundreds of faces staring at them, he knows he might have someone willing to bend to his will. Then it's a matter of finding the right pace—one that allows people to enjoy themselves but moves fast enough that the audience keeps to a joint rhythm.

A standard hypnotism session starts with something called an induction, in which the hypnotist paints a picture of a place or series of events meant to relax the subject: a flight of stairs, a long hallway, maybe a slowly rising balloon. The idea is to guide the person to push himself deeper and deeper into a trance. For many, this is the crucial moment when one little slipup can break the spell. When I tried to hypnotize a friend last year, it was the induction that sank me. I just couldn't find the right pace or words to make her forget herself. For

Newton, in addition to being effective, the induction has to be fast and entertaining.

Once hypnotized, some people struggle to remain so while others seem to go ever deeper. Those in the latter group not only make good patients but also make for a good show. In 1992, Newton convinced a group of hypnotizable people that they were eating apples when they were actually eating raw onions. It was so effective he even started an argument among the volunteers about what was in their hands!

Newton admits that the stage hypnotism world is littered with amateurs who don't know what they are doing and can even harm their subjects. But few people are as skilled at inductions as a good stage hypnotist. Hypnosis is as much an art as a science. Newton is well versed in psychology, especially in the psychology of group dynamics. Although he takes on a few hypnotherapy clients, he makes no secret of the fact that he is first and foremost a showman: His job is to hijack human behavior and use it to put on a good show. Sometimes that involves inducing a trance. But just as often it means using our herd mentality—our powerful inclination not to let down the people around us. In other words, just as with placebos, hypnosis can be enhanced with peer pressure.

Newton tends to see hypnotists everywhere around him—for instance, in military parades where soldiers march in lockstep and onlookers cheer on cue. He says one of the best hypnotists he's ever seen is Tony Robbins, perhaps the world's most famous motivational speaker, celebrated for his boundless energy and rock star–like persona. Robbins has a dedicated, almost cultlike following. Participants of his seminars often report feeling energized and ready to change their life afterward. Newton says it's not hard to spot his secret.

"He's using the oldest stage hypnotism trick in the book," he says. "He tells people when to stand, when to sit. He tells people when to high-five the person next to you, when to shake hands, when to hug the person next to you. When to pump your fist in the air shouting, 'Yes, yes, yes!' From there it's only one tiny little step away from telling people what to do, to what to think."

Newton observes that kneeling, praying, and chanting in unison is pretty much the script for mass hypnosis. In this light, it's easier to understand the power of everything from Nazi Germany to TV evangelists to boy bands like One Direction. They're all bringing people under their hypnotic spell. Newton tells me about the time 15 years ago when he went to see the American TV evangelist Benny Hinn: "Right from the word 'go,' I was one step ahead of him. In the audience, I knew exactly what he was going to do next, what he was going to say next. 'You will feel this tremendous power of the Holy Spirit. It will be uplifting. Some people will experience a tingling.' He's describing hypnosis."

Many religions, from Christianity to Sufism to Buddhism, employ some form of group trance (which is ironic, since many religions lump hypnosis in with satanic or occult practices). Singing, dancing, and chanting in unison, be they for healing or simply for getting in touch with a higher power, rely on the element of trance. And although it's true they can be used to manipulate people, trances (whether in a group or all alone) can also open a portal through which we can tinker with our expectations. Far from its alter ego as a cheap stage trick, hypnosis can be a powerful tool for healing.

● ● ●

Perhaps no one knows this better than David Patterson and Mark Jensen at the University of Washington in Seattle, two of the nation's leading experts on hypnosis. It may not be the sexiest field for modern scientists, but for Patterson and Jensen it's too seductive to ignore. "It's a very real phenomenon that no one can seem to explain,"

Patterson tells me. "I just can't wrap my brain around the fact it's actually happening and I don't know how it happens."

Patterson is the polar opposite of the stereotypical Svengali hypnotist. Laid-back and affable, he is quick to smile and speaks with a quiet, halting voice. He reminds me more of a kindly uncle than of a mind-bending magician. He's accustomed to dubious looks and snickering from people when he brings up his job, and occasionally wonders if he shouldn't just choose a more mainstream topic to study. But then something happens that blows his mind and sucks him back in.

Take a lecture on hypnotism and pain control at a burn unit that he gave at Vanderbilt University in the 1990s. The doctors had been skeptical. When Patterson offered to demonstrate his technique on one of them, they recommended that he try it on one of the patients, a young man Patterson described as "angry at the world" who had burns covering more than half his body. It is almost impossible to describe the agony of serious burns over large portions of the body. Several doctors I've interviewed say it is the worst pain a human being can experience. Every time a nurse tried to remove this patient's bandages to wash his wounds, he screamed and writhed in pain, despite a stream of powerful drugs.

This was the patient Patterson had been asked to treat. The young man scoffed at him, saying that he couldn't be hypnotized. Eventually he agreed to try it but seemed intent on doing the opposite of what he was told. So during the hypnosis, Patterson suggested he would become increasingly tense. As if on cue, the man did the opposite and became relaxed. Within a few minutes, he slipped easily into a deep, peaceful trance as nurses removed the bandages and rubbed sponges over his raw sores. (Patterson showed me a video from a similar case, and I can attest to this effect.)

Another time, in 1996, Patterson met a patient who had come in to the emergency room with—there's no delicate way to put this—a rusty ax in his neck. The doctors had saved the man after this terrible accident, but in the process he developed meningitis and had to have painful spinal taps regularly. By this time, Patterson was working as a hypnotist at the University of Washington hospital and was frantically running between patients. He had little time to hypnotize him, so he set to work fast.

"He was yelling and screaming," Patterson tells me. "I literally had five minutes. So I said, 'When the nurses touch you on the shoulder to roll you over, you'll go into a trance.'" For most people, a lightning-fast induction followed by a suggestion wouldn't work. But Patterson got lucky. The patient turned out to be highly hypnotizable. Afterward, when a nurse touched him, the man who had been screaming in pain suddenly became limp and malleable. "They would roll him over and he would become flaccid and just wouldn't feel anything," Patterson says. "He was totally conscious and had this goofy look on his face."

As with the tale of F. T. Moore, the young British boy with the horrifying skin disease, stories like this can prompt us to wonder why there isn't a hypnotist on staff at every hospital. But suggestibility isn't easy to prescribe.

"If you see ten patients, there'll be two of them where the hypnosis will make your jaw drop," Patterson says. "And then you are all excited. But you try it with another person and it's just not that dramatic. That's one of the maddening things about hypnosis."

True, only 10 percent of the population tends to respond strongly to the practice, but most only respond reasonably, or fairly, well. Also, hypnotists vary greatly in how well they ply their trade. Voice, speech rhythm, and timing can mean the difference between success and failure. Finding the right imagery to induce hypnosis is tough, and finding the right kind of story to make the suggestion really stick is even tougher. And even if a hypnotist gets the voice, pacing, and storytelling, he has to adapt well on the fly and follow his gut as to what is resonating with the patient. This makes it almost impossible to standardize an experiment. Imagine Sir Isaac Newton measuring the speed of a falling object, but Earth's gravity keeps changing. That's what it's like studying hypnosis.

Nevertheless, Patterson and his research partner Mark Jensen have made considerable strides by examining the neural underpinnings of a hypnotic trance. Jensen offers to show me one of the tools he uses in his work, called electroencephalography, or EEG, which measures electricity in the brain. Individual neurons are constantly generating electrical pulses as they transmit information from the body to the brain and around the brain itself. Occasionally, large groups of neurons will actually coordinate these pulses into a sort of rhythmic pattern, similar to an audience doing a wave in a stadium.

That's a little like what our brain cells seem to do, except with electricity. Using electrical sensors attached to the outside of the skull, scientists can listen for these broad electrical rhythms (called oscillations) of electricity caused by wide swaths of neurons working in concert. Keep in mind, though, that the brain isn't a single stadium, but rather 1.2 million interlocking stadiums at once. So the EEG may pick up many different interlocking elements at once: a sports cheer, an audience sing-along at a heavy metal concert, the national anthem, an orchestra tuning up.

To make matters more complicated, because the sensors are on the outside of your head, people like Jensen can measure only the outer parts of the brain. That makes the stadium even harder to hear. "The Rolling Stones are in town, but you don't have a ticket," he says. "So you are standing outside the stadium. It's very loose. You don't know what, exactly, you're hearing, but you can tell if they are singing a ballad or a rock song."

Amazingly, even with all these barriers, when scientists listen to multiple places in the brain, a neurological picture of hypnosis begins to emerge. For instance, although to people experiencing them meditation and hypnosis can feel very similar, they create very different scenarios. The "stadium chant" that many parts of your brain participate in during meditation is measurably slower than in daily life. And with hypnosis, it becomes even slower. About the only way to get brain rhythms slower than those during hypnosis would be to fall into a coma.

To demonstrate what this feels like, Jensen does a little experiment with me. In a drab, windowless room near his office, a student places a few EEG electrodes around the left side of my skull and a set of headphones over my ears. Jensen tells me to clear my mind, to just relax—a sort of self-hypnosis. As I attempt to do so, his student watches my brain waves begin to roll across her screen. Specifically, she is looking at my alpha and theta waves. Alpha waves—about 8 to 12 hertz (electric waves that pulse 8 to 12 times per second)—prevail when we are relaxed or just closing our eyes. Theta (4 to 8 hertz) commonly arise when we are drowsy or lost in thought. And the slowest, delta waves (0 to 4 hertz), happen when we are asleep or in a coma.

I can almost hear all the tiny neurons in my brain switching from their normal frenetic, random chatter to a rhythmic chanting. Whenever I'm doing a good job—below a certain threshold of theta waves—my headphones play a soothing New Age tune (it sounds like Enya and makes me even more relaxed). When my neurons are generating delta waves, I hear the soothing sounds of the ocean. And when both rhythms rise above their thresholds, I hear music soothingly paired with waves crashing.

But as soon as a thought pops into my mind, they stop. It's a horribly frustrating process. I sit, clear my mind, and try to create that dull, almost throbbing buzz you feel in your brain when you are thinking of nothing at all. And the music plays and the waves crash. And for a few seconds, it's perfect. Then I think, "This is going well," and they cut out.

What I didn't know was that every time I got deep enough to hear the waves and music, Jensen's student moved up the threshold of when I'd hear the theta waves, so that I had to be even more relaxed to hear them. I heard the music, the student raised the bar, the music cut out, and I went deeper, ever in search of that pleasant wave-music combination. By the end, I almost felt that I could turn on my delta and theta waves at will.

It's a good trick. Jensen uses this exercise as a training tool for subjects to master the use of brain waves to decrease pain, in much the same way that Kirsch had taught me to trick myself into holding down my leg so that I could remember what a basic form of suggestibility felt like.

Jensen's work suggests that theta and alpha waves may be key to pain relief. When going about our daily activities, the brain generally uses the much faster beta and gamma waves (up to 100 pulses per second). This is especially true when we're in pain, which usually goes hand in hand with anxiety and stress. Thus, if hypnosis and meditation can trigger slower brain waves, those waves may replace the faster patterns and thus replace the perception of pain. (This has nothing to do with the brain chemicals Tor Wager looks at. Just as there is more than one way to examine a roaring stadium, there is more than one way to look at a brain.) The implications for helping millions of people in chronic pain are enormous.

This conclusion led Jensen to a fascinating study. He looked at the brains of 20 patients before and after they experienced some relief from pain through both hypnosis and meditation. He found that people who naturally had high levels of theta waves—in other words, people with naturally relaxed, slower electrical activity—experienced a great deal of pain relief from hypnosis. Meanwhile, people with busy, overactive minds benefited the most from meditation, which slows their buzzing brains down to a crawl.

"Meditation takes care of a problem that you have. Hypnosis builds on a skill," Jensen says animatedly. "It's capitalization or compensation. Are you capitalizing on a strength or are you compensating for a weakness? It looks like meditation is compensating for a weakness, and hypnosis capitalizes on a strength."

Studies suggest that having a busy mind can limit a person's ability to manage pain. Imagine pain management as a skill, like running or weight lifting. According to Jensen, hypnosis is a little like taking an already strong sprinter to the gym and pushing her to a whole new level. Meditation is more like what happens when a couch potato, who has never worked out a day in his life, drastically changes his eating habits and starts running every day.

If Jensen is right, his research will back up much of what scientists have suspected for many years: Hypnosis is not a placebo or a trick of the mind that releases the brain's inner medicine cabinet. And it's not akin to distraction, which uses the brain's need to focus as a way to cloak the pain. By this line of reasoning, hypnosis may be an exotic brain state that directly accesses expectation and perception—a little like turning off all the software in your computer and accessing its basic coding. Except a bit more complicated.

● ● ●

After I've wrestled with my theta and alpha waves, it's time for me to get hypnotized. For that I go back to David Patterson's office at the University of Washington. With me is my friend and assistant, Liz Neely, who is there as much out of curiosity as to help me. Clearly she wants to try hypnosis too. But Patterson's time is valuable and she's not the one writing a book about suggestibility, so I give her the video camera and tell her to take a backseat and film the whole thing. Patterson begins by asking me about my family and then asks what complaint I'd like to address. I tell him about a pain I have in my arm and ask if he can focus on that. He seems a little disappointed, as chronic muscle pain usually takes a long time to treat with hypnosis. But he agrees to give it a shot as I sit down in an extremely comfortable chair in his office.

Hypnosis is all about suggestion, telling a story that captures the imagination and addresses the outcome you want to create. ("One of the ways to really engage people is storytelling," Patterson had told me. "You know Garrison Keillor and *Prairie Home Companion?* He's probably the best hypnotist who's ever lived.") But this is incredibly hard to do without breaking the "spell." If you stumble or lose your train of thought during the induction, or say something odd even once, the patient may notice and come out of the trance. I like to think I tell a pretty good story and am a smooth talker, but I'm a bumbling child next to David Patterson. (A few months before, I had tried to hypnotize a friend of mine, using a script Patterson had given me, but was a miserable failure. If you'd like to see if you can do any better, find the same induction in the appendix.)

In conversation, Patterson has a charming, self-deprecating sense of humor but stumbles and mumbles a little and, like many scientists, is easily distractible. As I sit down in his office, I can't imagine him hypnotizing anyone. But as he starts his induction he is instantly transformed. His voice becomes calm, confident, and as smooth as silk. Patterson begins by asking me to imagine my right arm is as light as a feather. He describes it filling with helium and lifting off my body. I try to imagine it but feel self-conscious, even a little silly. I want the treatment to magically lift my arm, but I don't want to lift it just to pretend I'm being hypnotized. And of course, these busy thoughts again keep me from relaxing.

He reaches out, lifts my hand, and sees that it isn't working. Without missing a beat, he changes tactics. Now, he says, my arm is as heavy as lead, planting itself into my leg. Dutifully, I imagine my arm planted into my leg like a lead weight. From there he launches into a 30-minute circular monologue. He begins integrating his treatment into a story meant to capture my attention and treat my pain.

He touches on multiple topics ranging from the pain in my arm to images of me floating in space, a feeling of freedom and peace, my father's arm injuries from playing baseball, and the need to separate my inquisitive mind from a relaxed one. His logic seems not to go anywhere yet continues forward, spinning around itself, repeating ideas while moving in no particular direction. I have trouble tracking it, which is the point, since I soon start to relax. But still, I struggle to enter a hypnotic trance. I imagine myself floating in space, starless but adorned with yellow and red nebulae that pass me as I fly by. It feels nice, but every few seconds I start wondering whether I'm hypnotized, which breaks the spell, and I have to start over.

In the end, I don't appear to be terribly hypnotizable. Patterson later says I am probably around a 3 out of 12 on the Stanford Hypnotic Susceptibility Scale. It comes as a bit of a disappointment. A few months before, I would have been proud of myself—feeling as if I had resisted the temptations of a wicked sorcerer, as if my failure to be hypnotized was some kind of superpower. But now that I understand the formidable power of hypnosis, it just feels like failure.

That's not to say I felt nothing. It's true, I wasn't in a trance. I didn't walk like a chicken or cry spontaneously. But I did feel a deep sense of relaxation. And when Patterson tried to pull me out of the treatment, I resisted. I was fully aware of myself; I just didn't want to open my eyes. I'm among those who used to think that people who are placebo prone or who easily fall into trances are somehow gullible. But Jensen flips that observation on its end. He thinks highly hypnotizable people are not only skilled but also "talented."

"It's a vulnerability and a real skill," he says. "It's not personality; it's just this ability of the brain to shift states and do things. And we take advantage of it with hypnosis by focusing people's attention on that ability." He pauses. "What are you telling yourself about yourself? If you have more hypnotic talent, our hypothesis is that the things you tell yourself are more strongly impactful."

By that reasoning, I am not talented. After I stand up, I can tell Patterson isn't satisfied. He looks at Liz as she turns off the camera, and his eyes seem to narrow. "Would you like to try?" he asks her.

In many ways, Liz and I are very similar people: happy-go-lucky, friendly, curious. That's probably how we became friends and why we've stayed that way. But there is an openness about her that I don't have. She's at the center of gatherings, where I might be just as happy lurking around the edges. (And, interestingly, she has a lot more white visible around her eyes.)

Perhaps Patterson sees this, or maybe he's just lucky. He takes her through a similar induction process, and almost from the beginning, Liz slips into a much deeper level of hypnosis than I had. When Patterson suggests that her arm is as light as a balloon, her arm lifts in the air as if attached to strings. When he tells her to lower it slowly back to her thigh, her arm drops so slowly that it seems as if it will never actually touch her leg. To look at her, I might have assumed that she was in some kind of trance, a hidden world unknowable to the average person, where she watched herself from a distance like a ghost. But she's totally conscious and in control of all her thoughts.

"I was just wondering why my hand hadn't touched my leg yet. It was as if my hand was kind of going through my leg," she says afterward.

Try it: Close your eyes, lift your hand off the table or your leg, and then slowly—ever, ever so slowly—lower it back down. Chances are that you will think your arm should have touched down long before it actually does. This, it turns out, is a big part of hypnosis: using tricks to create the sense that you are hypnotized, so that soon enough, you are.

Before leaving Jensen and Patterson's laboratory, I take a few minutes to see the team's new virtual-reality hypnosis software. Patterson, Jensen, and a third researcher/ace computer programmer, Hunter Hoffman, have been working on this idea for decades. If it works, it would make hypnotism much more feasible for scientists. One of the key problems with studying hypnosis is the imbalance in ability. Just as some patients are better at going under than others, some hypnotists are better at putting people under. It's hard to create a large-scale study when two of the main factors vary wildly from person to person. But if a computer program could work reasonably well, you could standardize half the equation. Just hook a patient up to the headgear, turn on the recording, and—bam!—instant pain relief.

The only problem is that virtual-reality hypnosis doesn't work that well. I'd seen an earlier version of Hoffman's program a few years earlier, and it was underwhelming. The viewer drifted into a snowbank and down into a snowy world. It's highly effective as a tool for distraction (like a video game that makes you forget your pain for a while), but it's not hypnotic. The shapes were blocky and the world was a little bland.

So I'm not all that excited to see the updated version—but we go along, just to be polite. The goggles aren't working, so Liz and I each stand in front of a simple computer screen, which isn't nearly as effective as a set of immersive virtual-reality goggles. Patterson's voice starts up over the computer's speaker. Instead of a snowbank, the screen shows an elegant computer-generated stream hemmed in by rocks and trees, and mountains beyond. It's very pleasant.

Then the viewer begins moving slowly down the stream past boulders and turns and shallow pools, as Patterson's voice slowly counts from 1 to 10, with each number flying toward the screen as he goes. I am fascinated, especially by the cool, blue water. It ripples rhythmically as the rocks pass beneath. And the edges of the stream gently undulate by. So gently. And easy.

Suddenly, I'm shaken awake by the noise of someone dumping a pile of electronics into a box and dragging it away. I realize that for a moment there I had nearly gone completely under. Then I look over at Liz. She's standing 10 feet away from her computer screen, leaning against the wall and looking pale.

"I had to move; I was about to pass out," she says meekly.

By the time the video got to about the number 7, Liz had felt her neck and shoulders slowly relax and then her hands went numb and tingly. Worried that she might fall over, she retreated to the back wall. All because of a video.

I didn't feel hypnotized, but there's no question this version is an improvement over the last. It's hard to say why for sure—I think it's that wonderfully undulating water. When Patterson had tried to hypnotize me before, it felt like an effort to keep a mental picture in my head. It was so much easier to just stare at the river and let my mind go.

For now, the track record for digital hypnosis still lags behind that administered by a real person. But without a doubt, digital hypnosis is coming.

● ● ●

I turned out to be a less-than-talented hypnotic subject. Does that make me feel like a big tough guy whose mind is impenetrable to suggestion? No, it makes me feel disappointed. Liz has so many more options open to her now that she knows she's hypnotizable. Pain relief, easing anxiety, quitting a bad habit—all these things become easier for hypnotizable people who can find a decent hypnotist.

So in the end, what can we say about hypnosis? It's not a placebo, and it's certainly not magic. But it is a powerful way to access expectation. A placebo says, "Take this amazing thing and it will make you feel better." It's a promise for the future. A hypnotic suggestion says, "Floating along this stream, you suddenly feel better," which is a promise for right now. Which one is better? Which one taps into your expectation more effectively and permanently? That's a question that will take many more hours in comfortable chairs listening to the calm, suggestive voice of a good hypnotist to unravel.

In the meantime, there are plenty of hypnotists out there who are as good as, if not better than, anyone I talked to. People who can—if you are sufficiently talented—take you on a journey of relaxation and relief from all kinds of maladies. Or, if you're uncomfortable with the more formal process, there are plenty of techniques out there to hypnotize yourself, not to mention some pretty amazing virtual-reality hypnosis tools that will be hitting the shelves in the future.

But there is one thing that hypnosis should never do. A type of suggestion—hypnotic or otherwise—that can ruin lives and even put innocent people in prison. If placebos are suggestions based in your future and hypnosis a suggestion for the present, then what would be a suggestion that affects your past? There is one. And it can be the most dangerous suggestion of all.

CHAPTER SIX

Satan Worshippers, Aliens, *and* Other Memories *of* Things That Never Happened

There are lots of people who mistake their
imagination for their memory.

—Josh Billings

I N MARCH 1988, RESIDENTS OF THE SMALL TOWN of Stuart, Florida, were gripped by what can only be described as mass hysteria. Law enforcement officers had discovered a secret satanic cult being run out of the local Montessori preschool. There were tales of dark hooded figures, bizarre blood ceremonies, and the ritualistic rape of children.

Evidence for this secret cult of child molesters came from none other than the children themselves—a decade later. Many of these remembered acts were so hideous, so barbaric, that the victims had buried the memories deep within their psyche, uncovering them only under intensive hypnosis. After hours of these sessions, psychologists and law enforcement officers were able to retrieve long-buried memories of bizarre ceremonies, torture, and the worst sexual violations imaginable. Psychologists flooded into town to uncover more debauchery and interview and save these innocent children.

"It got to be the kind of thing where every other storefront in the town had a new child psychologist," said resident Carol MacMillan. "I mean, it was a cottage industry for recovered memories."

The more psychologists and law enforcement dug down, the more instances of ritual abuse they turned up. Pretty soon, they had collected more than 60 testimonies of horrendous torture and sexual deviance. The community went ballistic. Some residents attended town meetings armed with handguns hunting for satanists, while others planted listening devices in classrooms and searched for mass graves on the school grounds. "It was like Salem all over again," one parent recalled.

As a result of the children's testimony, police arrested James Toward, the owner of the preschool, and his office manager. Then they investigated Toward's wife, who also worked at the school. The case against her was weak, so the lawyers and psychologists reached out to a new round of kids to find new details that might implicate her. Among them was Carol MacMillan's daughter, an anxious little blond girl named Kristin Grace Erickson. Erickson was 12 years old at the time she was hypnotized. She understood from the doctors and other adults in town that her preschool teacher and his colleagues had done some terrible things—and could do more if people didn't do something to help. She trusted the doctors who brought her into an interview room, put her under hypnosis, and began asking questions.

As we've learned, you can't make people do something against their will under hypnosis, but a subject can become highly suggestible. Erickson recalls that a psychologist started asking probing questions about her experience at the preschool when she was a toddler. Initially, she had pleasant memories of the place, with its caring staff and occasional campfire sleepover. But after a few sessions, she began remembering bizarre rituals and being placed on a table where she was probed by cult members.

"I said that I saw a snake get killed and sliced down the side and that we had to drink its blood. And that there were people in hoods around a fire," she says.

The psychologist seemed pleased and pushed for more details, especially about Toward's wife. After the session was over, Erickson felt odd. She knew that by telling these people what had happened she was protecting other children who might be in danger. But she wasn't sure that what she had said was completely true. The memory felt funny, like a lie. So she timidly suggested to the psychologist that she might have made the whole thing up. "No," she remembers him saying, "that's just what it feels like. It really happened."

For the next 15 years or so, Erickson lived with the knowledge that she had been molested by a satanic cult masquerading as a Montessori preschool. Then, while living in San Francisco in her 20s, she decided to experiment with a sensory-deprivation tank—a chamber half filled with tepid water and impervious to sound or light. Crawl into one and you feel as if you are floating silently in the blackest space. For decades, people have used this extreme sort of quiet blackness as a sort of forced meditation.

At first she felt nothing but silence and boredom. But in the last few minutes, Erickson had an epiphany. She realized that something from her childhood hypnosis therapy was haunting her, and that she needed to come to terms with it. Soon afterward, she looked up Alan Tesson, one of the psychologists involved in the case, and was shocked to learn that 10 years after the investigations, he had been sued for implanting false memories in one of his patients.

What the hell is a false memory, she wondered? A memory that's not true is called a lie.

What Erickson didn't know was that her case had occurred in the middle of the so-called the Satanic Panic of the 1980s and '90s. A 1992 FBI report noted during this period "hundreds of victims alleging that thousands of offenders are abusing and even murdering tens of thousands of people as part of organized satanic cults—and there is little or no corroborative evidence."

Today, scientists understand that what caused a nationwide panic and the imprisonment of dozens of people wasn't a conspiracy of pedophiles but an interesting glitch in the human mind: specifically, how we create memories.

●　●　●

You might assume that when you take in the world around you, your eyes and ears act like video cameras and tape recorders. That what you are seeing and hearing is what *is:* a park bench looking out over a wooded hillside, the furniture in your living room, the words on this page.

But in reality, your eyes and ears are taking light and sound and turning them into electrical signals to the brain, which then has to construct a version of what is being seen that makes sense. To do that, your brain has to make assumptions and take shortcuts, and it sometimes makes mistakes. Optical illusions, blind spots, and hallucinations all demonstrate how your brain can misinterpret what it's seeing—to potentially very confusing and dangerous ends. Brain injuries like visual agnosia, an impairment popularized by Oliver Sacks in his book *The Man Who Mistook His Wife for a Hat,* cause a person with perfect eyesight to be unable to recognize the objects he sees. And even if your brain works perfectly, a talented magician can fool you simply by toying with your attention and expectation.

Just as vision is not a simple camera, memories aren't like the CDs collecting dust in the corner of your attic. Like sight, memory is an integrated constructive process that is constantly refining itself—rebuilding, restructuring, and finding shortcuts. And, just as optical illusions do, your memory can play tricks on you.

When administering a placebo, the trick is to convince the subject that there is something in the pill that's not actually there. In hypnosis, it's to replace reality with a story or imagery that changes how the mind perceives, say, pain. Both are suggestions: This pill has powerful drugs in it; your arm isn't in searing pain—it's cool as a lake. Well, memory is equally responsive to suggestion. Not the suggestion of what's *about* to occur, but of what already has occurred.

To understand this, it helps to know a little about how memory works. Broadly speaking, your memories are created in three stages: encoding, consolidation, and retrieval. *Encoding* happens just as an event is occurring—that moment when you find yourself paying attention to something. All day, every day, your brain is taking all the sights, smells, and sounds around you, making sense of them, and storing them in your short-term memory: *I am putting my keys in the green dish by the door; that bird on the tree looks like a black-capped chickadee; I think I smell something burning*—these are all observations that your brain turns into memories. Any one of them could become part of a memory that you will carry for the rest of your life, depending on the next stage.

Consolidation is the transfer from short-term to long-term memory over the course of hours, weeks, or even years. It's a complicated and somewhat mysterious process whereby certain synapses (the gaps between brain cells) become sensitive, and several neurons begin firing in concert. Repetition of information certainly helps, as do stress hormones (which is why we remember stressful situations so vividly) and deep sleep (many scientists think dreaming is connected to consolidation).[14] Think of it as a mental filing system. At the end of the day, your mind sifts through all the memories it's made that day *(where my keys were before I left the house; whether that was a chickadee or a nuthatch)*, and moves only the important ones *(my moronic roommate accidentally lit the kitchen on fire)* into long-term memory.

The last step in creating memories is *retrieval*—that moment when you actually remember something. You might say that retrieving a memory is different from creating one. After all, you are just going through your metaphorical filing cabinet and pulling out a photo, right? No. Memory isn't static like photos. It's more like reassembling a picture from jigsaw pieces or making a photocopy of a picture and then looking at it. The point is that memory *retrieval* is its own sort of creation. And each time you make a copy, it looks a little different—a little more blurry and faded. So eventually you have to take a permanent marker and fill in some of the edges to make it appear sharper.

Simply put, a false memory is an error in one of these steps. And once that error occurs, it's almost impossible to correct. Take, for instance, a classic study by the legendary psychologist and memory expert Ulric Neisser. The morning after the explosion of NASA's space shuttle *Challenger* in 1986, Neisser took a poll of where his students were when they first heard about it. Almost three years later he ran

---

14 Interestingly, among the symptoms of post-traumatic stress disorder (PTSD) are nightmares and insomnia as patients relive horrendous memories again and again. PTSD is also often correlated with people who suffer from sleep problems, such as sleep apnea. But what if patients' inability to sleep was not a result of PTSD but rather the cause of it? That, without the crucial time to file them, the memories are left in a sort of mental limbo, torturing the person until they get put away. When you think of it that way, PTSD might not be an anxiety or a stress disease but rather a type of sleep disorder.

the poll again; almost all the answers had changed in some way. Several people had even placed themselves in totally different circumstances and refused to believe that the accounts they had written two years before were correct.

This in itself is startling and a little disconcerting. But most of the memory changes seemed to follow a pattern that made them (a) more dramatic and (b) more in line with a coherent narrative. This is at least in part the result of the so-called flashbulb memory effect, in which red-letter events such as the assassination of John F. Kennedy, the *Challenger* explosion, and the attacks of 9/11 tend to be retold many times—and with each telling, become slightly different.

Sound familiar? What else requires a narrative that resonates well in order to change reality from what is to what we expect? I could easily be describing placebos or hypnosis. Expectation clouded by suggestion and good storytelling. As with placebos, false memories are tied to our brains, which are prediction machines, and to how we make sense of the world around us. As you're walking down the street, you can't constantly be checking to see if the pavement will suddenly turn into baked potato or puppies will start to fall from the sky. So your brain sets up certain expectations and then sets them aside. *The ground is hard. Puppies are mostly earthbound.*

To navigate the world the brain needs memories to know what it should and shouldn't do. Daniel Schacter, a psychologist and the author of the seminal *The Seven Sins of Memory* and many other acclaimed books on the subject, says the brain uses the past to imagine what will happen in the future. (This is not the first time we've seen this. Similarly, our memory of pain relief from taking an aspirin heightens our expectation when taking one in the future.) From his Harvard office overlooking Boston, he explains that in many ways, the brain treats the future and the past the same way. For instance, imagining the future and remembering the past use many of the same networks and occupy similar real estate in the brain. As we age and our recollection of the past fades, so, too, does our ability to imagine the future with any degree of detail.

"Memory really is the version we told most recently," Schacter says. "That function—flexible use of the past to think about the future—is something that may make memory error prone."

In *The Seven Sins of Memory*, Schacter points out that our brains' memory weaknesses actually derive from their strengths. Strong emotion helps create memories that are easy to access later, but those same memories can develop into phobias or even debilitating PTSD. That same ability to use the past to predict the future can cause occasional errors in memories of the past.

This is not the same as forgetting, Schacter says. When you forget something, you *know* you've forgotten it. But with a false memory, you may not even realize what's happened unless you come across evidence that your memory is wrong. It's not really our fault, I suppose; it's just that we are accustomed to accepting what our memory tells us. Schacter is careful to clarify that memory and imagination are not the same thing. But he says they definitely hang together. Thus it's not hard to see how a person in a state of deep, suggestible relaxation might let his imagination go, and then interpret what he sees as a true memory. And indeed, one of Schacter's seven sins is our old friend suggestibility.[15]

● ● ●

Daniel Schacter was one of the first scientists to look seriously at the nature of false memories, but the person who brought them into

_____

15 The other six are transience, blocking, misattribution, bias, persistence, and my personal favorite, absent-mindedness.

the global spotlight was University of California, Irvine, psychologist Elizabeth Loftus. Her research over the past three and a half decades has upended everything we thought we knew about this phenomenon.

After graduating from Stanford in 1974, Loftus began working for the U.S. Department of Transportation, examining eyewitness accounts of accidents. She noticed that when estimating the speed of cars involved in crashes, witnesses answered differently depending on how the question was phrased. The highest estimates went to those trying to guess the speeds of two cars that "smashed" into each other. Second highest were for cars that "hit" each other, and the lowest were for the ones that "made contact" with each other. Loftus began to wonder how deep this "memory contamination," as she calls it, goes.

In the mid-1970s, this led to one of her most famous sets of experiments. People viewed slides of a red Datsun passing a stop sign and then smacking a pedestrian. The experimenters asked the subjects a number of questions, some of which are a little misleading, like, "Did another car pass the red Datsun while it was stopped at the yield sign?" The subject thinks for a moment and then says to herself, *No, I definitely didn't see any other cars next to that yield sign.* And voilà, the sign has changed in their minds.

You see, as the subjects are trying to make sense of what is happening in front of them, they are falling back on the frameworks in their brains, built over the course of their whole lives. And it turns out that sometimes the observed reality is more fluid than the preconceived story. *Was that a yield sign? Yeah, yeah—I think it was.* Many people think of memory as some kind of video, one that you can simply rewind to see what happened. In Hollywood films, when the hero needs to retrieve some piece of information from the past, he'll use a clever trick—guided imagery, hypnosis, maybe a magical steel drum that holds glowing blue memories—so he can go back and look for details he may not have seen the first time. It's a nice idea, but such hidden memories, if they exist, are extremely rare. More often, when you try to go back in time, your mind simply fills in the blanks with something that *seems* right, given the story it's trying to construct. We all have memories like this—things we're sure about and that we can see with our eyes closed—that just aren't true.

My favorite false memory is the one that opens this book. The story of my near miss with death as a baby became a legend in my family; while I was growing up, it fascinated me that I almost died and that God had saved me. I imagined what it would have been like, and asked my parents about it regularly. Today I can recall that fateful night with near-perfect clarity: the fear in my parents' eyes, the baby dying in their arms, even the gray dotted wallpaper. I can see it as if it were yesterday, and if you were to ask me for details about the room, I could provide them. The grandfather clock in the corner, the wooden table by the couch.

There are just three problems. First, the wallpaper wasn't gray; it was a bright yellow-orange. Second, I can see the baby in my mind's eye. The baby who was me. When I told Schacter about this, he pointed out that a few very old memories can occasionally change from a "field" memory (one where you are looking out from your own perspective) to an "observer" memory (one where you become an invisible person looking over what is happening). Scientists aren't exactly sure why this occurs, but there is some evidence to suggest that observer memories are less accurate than field memories. Third, and most important, a one-year-old isn't capable of forming long-term memories. But a young boy fascinated with an event in his past certainly can, retroactively. And so can an adult. Every time I was either told about that night or turned it around in my head, trying to imagine what it might have been like, how I might have felt, I was actually creating a rich picture of the events that looked a lot like a memory. Then, over time, as I thought back, not to the event but to the times I had thought about it, it actually *became* a memory. Even now, after talking to my parents and looking through old photos to confirm that indeed the gray wallpaper never existed, I can see the color of the wallpaper in my memory start to change.

After her traffic accident research, Loftus began focusing all her attention on this kind of corrupted memory. Over the years, she has managed to implant dozens of scenarios from people's childhoods that never actually happened. In one, she convinced a healthy segment of her subjects that they had once gotten lost in a mall as a child and their parents had been panicked until a kindly man in a jean jacket found them and returned them. To get the memory to stick, she used all her suggestive prowess (as with the yield sign), and added a new element by bringing in trusted family members to testify to the accuracy of the lost-kid narrative. Within weeks, about a quarter of her subjects remembered the event as real.

Once the memory was created, of course, people began filling in details of their own, just as I did with the wallpaper ("Oh yeah, he had boots and a shiny belt buckle!"). When critics suggested that perhaps Loftus had uncovered an actual memory of getting lost in a mall (apparently guys wearing jean jackets have saved hundreds of kids in malls over the years), she took up the challenge. She implanted memories in people that they had gone to Disneyland to meet Bugs Bunny. They posed for photos, shook his hand, some even got a lollipop.

Except that Bugs doesn't live in Disneyland. He's the property of Disney's archrival, Warner Bros. It's kind of like remembering having seen the pope perform morning prayers at the Great Mosque of

Algiers. No matter how bizarre or alien the scenario seems, there is someone out there who will believe it happened to them.

"We are almost at the point of having a recipe for how to do this," Loftus says. "A first step involves trying to make people feel something is *plausible*. In questionable therapy, people are told that many, many people have repressed memories and that you need to uncover them to feel better. That is a plausibility-enhancing message."

The second step, she says, is to create a sense of *recollection*. "Once people believe something could have happened to them or that it did happen, they may not have any kind of feeling of recollection. Then you engage them in imagination exercises where you put sensory details into this belief. And it starts to be experienced as a recollection." That's where the jean jacket and the image of Bugs Bunny come in.

At the same time that Loftus was conducting these tests, she began actively working as an expert witness and consultant in criminal court cases. Her testimony cast doubt on eyewitness reports, especially those that came about through hypnosis. She convinced dozens of juries that what one person thought had happened might not have been real.

Loftus found that false memories were littered across law enforcement, and that there are numerous ways a memory can be pushed on a witness. The hit Netflix series *Making a Murderer* demonstrated this perfectly in 2015 when it showed how a quiet teenager was bullied by police officers during an interrogation into remembering an event that may not have occurred. It's a circumstance that can also happen by accident. For instance, if you show a witness a string of black-and-white mug shots, plus one high school graduation picture in color, it's possible to create a memory around the color picture, just because it's different. Or if you show someone a lineup of mug shots and then take just one of those photos and put it into a different grouping, the witness can "recognize" that person and implant them into the crime scene.

In the cases Loftus consulted on, some of clients were guilty—for example, Ted Bundy[16] and Martha Stewart—and some were not. But over time, the notion that some memories might not be real (especially fantastical ones unearthed by hypnosis) took hold in academia and the courtroom. The debates that ensued between those who thought memories could be repressed by trauma and those who thought that most "repressed" memories were false or induced are known today as the "memory wars."

Eventually a certain pattern started forming in many inexplicable stories of abuse. An adult sees a therapist for anxiety or depression or maybe an eating disorder. Looking for a silver bullet to explain the problem, the therapist suggests hypnosis. (Sadly, good hypnosis instruction is hard to find, and plenty of places will teach you just enough to be dangerous. Responsible hypnotists like David Patterson take years to perfect their craft, learning to avoid specific words that might bias the subject or accidentally implant ideas.) Although repressed memories certainly could exist in theory (and indeed "dissociative amnesia," its technical name, is still listed in the latest version of the *Diagnostic and Statistical Manual of Mental Disorders*), they are difficult to study in the laboratory, and some experts assert that they don't exist at all.

There are very few documented examples of repressed memories. Loftus says there is simply no evidence that people can create amnesia through sheer terror, and that all the examples compiled in the 1990s could be explained in other ways. Often, she says, they are just false memories. Richard McNally, who has co-written books with Schacter, is equally skeptical that a person can somehow eradicate traumatic memories and then discover them again years later. He has a simpler

---

16 Loftus aided in Bundy's defense after his first arrest, before the public knew of his string of murders.

explanation, though: Maybe they just forgot. Very small kids might not even understand what's happening to them at the time. Only if they somehow remember the experience as an adult would they realize—and be traumatized by—what has been done to them.

For Kristin Grace Erickson, the realization that her childhood abuse had been a combination of overreaching psychologists and her overactive imagination was a bittersweet revelation. And the more she thought about it, the more she realized the similarities with events she had seen on television. "I had seen enough satanic movies—*Children of the Corn,* whatever—that I knew the kind of imagery they were looking for," she says.

Erickson remembers that she was trying to be helpful and that she believed her parents and the doctors unconditionally. Plus, she says, she enjoyed the attention. It's a similar story given by numerous child witnesses who have since recanted. Some have discovered their memories to be false; others knew they were lying from the beginning but just wanted to make the adults happy.

In one case from 1992, a detective asked a child witness if a defendant, the child's grandfather, had poured anything on her while abusing her. The child answered no. He asked again, this time asking if it had been a liquid. Again, no. Then the interviewer asked whether the defendant had poured oil or ketchup on her, and the child responded, "Ketchup." Despite a lack of physical evidence, the defendant, Bruce Perkins, was convicted and is still in prison today, steadfastly maintaining his innocence.

In another example almost too spectacular to believe, a woman who was hypnotized for depression and weight issues became convinced she had participated in the murder of her sister as part of her parents' satanic practices. Her sister, however, had died several years before the woman was even born. The memories had risen from her childhood curiosity with a dead sister she'd never met.

It's not clear how many innocent people are currently in prison because of false-memory testimony, but every year counties and states regularly quietly release supposed child molesters who have spent decades in prison based on the testimony of hypnotized children.

Erickson says that she was a troubled and anxious child, and the story that she had been molested in preschool gave her parents something to pin it on. As an adult, she's had difficult relationships with men, and when her brother had a baby, she didn't trust herself around her nephew for fear that somehow she would snap and suddenly become a child molester herself. Although she no longer believes she was abused in ritualistic fashion, she still has trouble trusting people and taking things at face value. After all, when you are told at 10 that you were abused by satanists and then realize at 25 that you weren't, it's hard to know what's real.

To make matters worse, many false memories possess a kernel of truth, hidden under layers of invention. For instance, Erickson says that she vaguely remembers a campout at the preschool with tents and sleeping bags and a huge campfire, built by James Toward, the school's owner. (Sure, having small kids camp out in a preschool playground is a little odd and maybe created an opportunity for parents to mistrust the school.) When she woke the next morning, she remembers that someone said a snake had ventured too close to the kids and that Toward had killed it. She never saw the snake but it was all very exciting at the time. These memories, she now thinks, were the seeds of an invented satanic ceremony around a fire with children drinking snake blood.

Trying to ease her guilt over her role in Toward's conviction, Erickson led an effort to get him released from prison. In the process she learned that he had been found guilty of statutory rape. He may not have probed children as a part of satanic rituals, but investigators did find he'd paid two underage boys in a poor, largely minority neighborhood for sex. (And although tens of millions of dollars went to the victims of supposed ritual abuse, not a penny went to the two kids Toward had actually abused.) Eventually, Toward—who was born in Europe—was released from prison under the condition that he leave the United States forever.

• • •

Scientists have been able to paint a rich picture of how false memories might function in the brain. They can form at any stage of memory making: during the initial encoding; during the consolidation into long-term memory; and during retrieval of the memory days, months, or years later. We know that in some people false memories can be just as powerful and even longer lasting than real memories. They also have a lot in common with "gist" or "fuzzy" memories. As opposed to the more specific "verbatim" memory ("My address growing up was 35 Grove Street"), a gist memory is based on semantics and occurs when you have a general idea of what happened but can't recall all the details ("That house was at the top of a massive hill"). In other words, a gist memory fits into a story that we tell ourselves to help us remember something.

There are several ways that scientists tinker with such memories. For instance, imagine seeing a list of words in different colors. "Basketball" is blue, "nitrogen" is green, "juice" is yellow, "net" is purple, "soccer" is red, and "sand" is black. Which color is juice? That's a verbatim memory. How many deal with a sports theme? That's a semantic, gist memory. The theory goes that the brain codes these two types of memories differently. And it turns out the gist category is easy to mess with. If I ask you whether "juice" is blue, there's a good chance you'll either remember correctly or confidently say that you don't remember. However, with a long enough list and enough other words meant to confuse you, I might be able to convince you that "volleyball" is on that list, because it fits in with the sports theme and because you saw "net" and "sand."[17]

This is why false memories are so powerful: They fit with the existing narrative so well that they seem plausibly true. It's fun—making you think I said "volleyball" when I really said "sand." But its value lies in allowing scientists to study the mechanisms of false memories in the laboratory. One of the challenges is how to spot a false memory. Surely it looks different from a real memory in the brain, right?

Some experts observe that on the surface, false memories don't contain as much detail as real memories do. Other studies conclude that false memories last longer than real ones. Still others have suggested that the emotions around false memories aren't as strong. But none of these has held up to repeated testing.

So far, no reliable trait has emerged as a way to spot false memories, so the search has shifted to brain imaging. Which, as you can imagine, is enormously difficult. Remember how hard it was to detect someone in pain by looking at a brain image? Imagine how hard it is to spot a lie when the person telling it doesn't even realize it's a lie. (Most lie detectors rely on subtle physiological changes—eye movement, pulse, skin conductivity—triggered by the knowledge that a person is lying. These triggers disappear when the subject doesn't know he's lying.) Scientists have spent years trying to see conscious deception in the brain. One technique even led to the development of a company (called No Lie fMRI), but in the end it still couldn't separate lies from background noise. So how are they supposed to separate a false memory?

Part of the difficulty arises from the fact that memory formation, with its three distinct stages, is involved in a lot of different parts of the brain. But what if there was a different way to approach the

---

17 This style of word suggestion testing is called the Deese–Roediger–McDermott paradigm, but other techniques use shapes, sounds, pretty much anything that people experience and remember.

question? What if, rather than trying to determine whether a given memory is real or not, we could find out whether a given person is prone to false memories?

Several studies have linked the very young and the very old to a propensity for false memories—which would explain some aspects of the phenomenon of recovered abuse memories. And yet a 2007 study from Great Britain showed that children are actually better at suppressing false memories during recall than adults are, demonstrating that it takes conscious energy for them to create such memories. Other experts have noted that very young kids don't make the inferences needed (such as, in one study, replacing a grapefruit with an orange). A small 2015 Canadian study—using memory games during a science fair magic show—found that kids do make false memories, and furthermore they are more likely to remember them while forgetting the true ones through something called retrieval-induced forgetting, which is the forgetting of one thing through remembering another, to purge false memories.

So maybe age isn't the key. Look at other factors: Some researchers have said false memories are linked to intelligence, education level, and "poor perceptual abilities." Others have said they are tied to working memory (the ability to hold on to relevant information as it's coming at you) and that a bad working memory indicates a propensity for false memories. My personal favorite ties a talent for false memories to an individual's level of hypnotizability. And although it would explain a lot about what happened to Erikson, the connection between false memories and race, age, intelligence, and hypnotizability are still pretty weak. Meanwhile, other researchers have found a link between false memories and intelligence, education level, and "poor perceptual abilities"—but none of those results have held up over time.

In 2015, a Spanish team, in a conclusion that will surprise no one, found that cannabis use encourages false memories. But what *was* surprising was that even after people stopped smoking weed, they remained prone to creating false memories, suggesting some kind of long-term changes to the brain's medial temporal lobe as a result of regular marijuana use. A similar effect, though perhaps in a different brain region, probably exists as a result of sleep deprivation.

It seems as if all these scientists are wandering about, rudderless. Brain imaging conferences today are littered with similar eclectic research into false memories. But we actually know more about the phenomenon than I am letting on.For one thing, we know that multiple regions of the brain—tied not only to memory but also to imagination, perception, and emotion—play roles in creating false memories. We know that errors can happen at any time in the process of making and recalling memories. We know that the emotional power and certainty of a false memory is just as strong as, if not stronger than, a real memory. And we know that no matter how immune we may think we are, anyone can have one. In one study, even people with the disorder hyperthymesia, which causes them to remember every event in their lives in painstaking detail, were susceptible to false memories at roughly the same rate as the rest of us.

In 2010, Elizabeth Loftus and a group of Chinese experts tested for more psychology-oriented traits like "fear of negative evaluation," "harm avoidance," "cooperativeness," "reward dependence," and "self-directedness" to see if any of them might predict the propensity for false memories. They found that no one trait predicted false memory production, but that certain combinations do. For instance, someone unfazed by danger or other people's negative opinions, yet highly cooperative and reward-driven, might be in the sweet spot for the propensity toward false memories. (Of course, we can't talk about reward-driven mentalities without thinking of dopamine, which drives that system.) But without knowing more about what mechanisms in the brain control false memories, we can't read too much into that yet.

Some might say the solution to imprecise personality tests is not to combine them with other equally vague measures. But as with Kathryn Hall's *COMT*-placebo work, this kind of thinking gets at a deeper truth: namely, that many parts of your mind and personality contribute to how suggestible you are.

In the end, a false memory—like a placebo response—is likely to be related to numerous conscious and unconscious brain processes. It is related to your personality, your worldview, perhaps your genetics, and even your mood on a particular day. And it is also dependent on authority. To get people to believe her "lost in the mall" scenario, Loftus had to recruit a subject's older family members to coax the person into remembering something that didn't happen. The same is true when looking at a police lineup. If the cops let slip which suspect they think is the perpetrator, the witness tends to shape his memory around that person.

Our expectations say as much about who we are and where we come from as they do about genetics, age, or brain chemistry. Suggestibility, it seems, is a collision of our brains, our bodies, and our individual histories that shape the stories we tell ourselves.

• • •

Of course, not all false memories deal with molestation, abuse, or crime. Scientist Richard McNally spent years looking at false memories and claims of childhood trauma similar to Erickson's and kept running into the same problem. Although it was unlikely that the elaborate satanic rituals had ever occurred, it was impossible to rule out the possibility that something—some kernel of true abuse—had happened. How can you understand false memories if there is a chance that some of the memories you are studying are true? So he turned to the next logical place to conduct memory research—little green men from outer space.

The nearest solar system to our own is Alpha Centauri, 4.37 light-years away. That might sound pretty close if you are a fan of *Star Trek*, but each light-year is about six trillion miles long. The Voyager 1 space probe, which was launched when I was about eight months old and has been rocketing away from us at roughly 39,600 miles an hour, has traveled less than two-tenths of *one percent* of one light-year.

Meanwhile, the nearest planet we have found to date that could sustain life, called Wolf 1061, is 13.8 light-years away. For a creature living there to visit us, it would have to break almost every law of physics and still endure an extremely long trip. It's a fair bet that after such a grueling journey, the last thing a space creature would want to do is quietly pick someone out of their bed and extract semen or eggs. At least that was McNally's assumption. Therefore, people who claim to have been abducted by aliens must have instead experienced some form of false memory.[18]

When you imagine someone who has been abducted by aliens, you probably envision a person in a tinfoil hat, alternatively whispering and screaming lines from David Lynch movies. But when McNally started this work, he was surprised to find that those who had professed to have this experience were "bright, articulate, pleasant, and seemingly sane." In fact, that's what grabbed his attention. Many (but not all) had uncovered their long-repressed memories through hypnosis. How could normal people have such abnormal beliefs?[19]

---

18 Of course, in science you can never prove a negative, especially one involving alien technology or interdimensional travel. But you have to start somewhere, and plenty of very solid science has begun with shakier assumptions than this.

19 As with the Laotians killed by their own fear (see chapter 4), many alien abductees suffer from some form of sleep paralysis. When a journalist suggested this to one of McNally's subjects, who suffered from sleep paralysis and hallucinations, McNally says the man said, "Believe me—they're different. You really have to have experienced both of them to know the difference."

In 2002, when McNally conducted an experiment at Harvard using lists of related words, he found that people claiming to have had contact with aliens were about twice as likely to form false memories as a control group (this was also the case in people with repressed memories). Interestingly, when they thought back on their experiences, they had many of the same bodily responses—sweating, arousal measured through the skin—as patients with PTSD. These are some of the same measures that Tor Wager saw when looking at placebo responses, and they can't be faked. In other words, the people's beliefs affected their bodies, in a way similar to the physical effects of those who had survived a harrowing experience. But that doesn't clinch it, according to McNally: "The vividness of their abduction memories generates the physiology hitherto attributable only to traumatic events," he says. "Vividness is not a guarantor of authenticity."

McNally and his students soon started looking at past-life regression—people who have had the experience of glimpsing themselves in a former life. As with those who had experienced satanic abuse, most of them had found their former lives through hypnosis, and McNally saw the same trends and the same suggestibility. Paul Simpson, a former hypnotherapist who performed such treatment and later realized (in 1993) that he'd been implanting false memories, says there are five types of experiences that are created by false memories and yet can become a central part of a person's life: abuse, satanic ritual abuse,[20] regression into the womb, alien abduction, and prior life trauma. Since then, he's counseled and interviewed hundreds of people who fell into these categories.

Simpson was struck by the similarity of these cases. Most subjects had sought help from a counselor for some personal problem, such

---

20 Which he separates from normal abuse because of its elaborate structure and the fact that it usually includes several generations of Satan-worshippers working together.

as depression or weight loss, and then been put into a trance—whether it was called hypnosis, eye-movement desensitization and reprocessing, or (among some Christian groups) Holy Spirit–inspired visions and guidance. He also noticed that the people who "remembered" satanic cults never overlapped with those who said they'd experienced alien abduction, and vice versa. If you were setting out to find alien abductees through hypnosis, wouldn't it make sense that you'd find at least a few satanic-ritual survivors? But no, researchers tend to find exactly what they are looking for. Indeed, a few experiments in the '90s even tested this notion by implanting memories in unsuspecting subjects. Sure enough, the best predictor for what the therapist found was what the therapist expected to find.

Aliens, satanic cults, murder, and mayhem—the world of false-memory research certainly is never boring. But it's not necessarily a bad thing to experience the occasional false memory. For one thing, McNally and a number of other researchers have found that people who say they've been subjected to UFO abductions and other experiences largely attributable to false memories also tend to be more creative, imaginative, and accepting of new ideas. False memories have been linked in several studies to the ability of "magical ideation," or magical thinking. Magical thinking, for its part, is thought to be tied to our old friend dopamine. People who score low on magical-ideation surveys often have trouble enjoying themselves, struggle to find meaning in life, and often battle depression.

Humans are not alone in creating false memories; pigeons, mice, and even bumblebees seem to have them.[21] That suggests false mem-

---

21 The last of these was discovered through a rather ingenious experiment. Biologists taught bees that a specific pattern on a flower contained nectar. So the next day, the bees knew exactly which one to return to. But over time they seemed to misremember the pattern and would first go to a similar one that they had never seen before.

ories may just be a part of how we think—a by-product of our innate ability to group things together by theme. As Schacter says, memories are a tool to help animals predict the future by using the past. And to do that, we humans have become experts at quickly grouping things together and creating patterns.

Think about a dog. What does a dog need to get out of a memory? Dogs are relatively clever, but they can't manage the impressive feats of memory that humans can. They need to know where the best bits of trash are in the neighborhood and where they buried that drumstick they didn't finish two days ago. Certainly they need to know where little Billy Jenkins lives because Billy likes to shoot dogs with his BB gun. Being social, they also need detailed memories about pack dynamics—who's on top, who they can push around.

But all these memories are tagged to emotional or sensory experiences. *Liked this. Didn't like that. This was delicious. That was scary.* They don't need perfect recall. The amount of effort their brains would need to create perfect memories of everything that happens to them just wouldn't be worth it.

Now imagine our ancient ancestors—those pre-humans who evolved increasingly complex brains with fuller, more detailed memories over millions of years. They could store food for the winter, construct complex hunting grounds, predict the movements of animals. They had highly complex social hierarchies and could remember details about other proto-humans they'd met 5, 10, 20 years before. They could also remember the details of the tools they built—how to do it right, how to do it better. But there was never a point at which they needed perfect accuracy. This is not to say that they had second-rate memories; it was just that they didn't require perfect recall. And who knows, maybe there was some advantage to being able to remember events the way you want to, rather than the way they actually happened. (Certainly it would have made you a lot more fun to sit around a fire with.)

Fast-forward to the 21st century. As with our ancient ancestors, we rely on our memories every day. *Where did I put my wallet? What's the country code for dialing Britain? When do I stop wearing white— Labor Day or Memorial Day? And seriously, where the hell did I put my wallet?!*

Most of the time, our memories are correct, leading us to think that what we remember is the way things actually were. Just like the dog trying to find that bone he buried, it's good enough. But it's not perfect—and it's certainly not a video archive.

● ● ●

In the end, we can't always trust what our memories are telling us. But that knowledge in itself can be powerful. Once you understand that people's memories are less videotape and more extended personal narrative, the world begins to make a little more sense. Autobiographies cease to be absolute truth and turn more to "some stuff that happened mixed with some stuff that probably didn't."

And no one is immune to this tendency. In February 2015, TV anchor Brian Williams lost one of the most prestigious journalism jobs in the country after retelling a story for the umpteenth time about having been shot at by a rocket-propelled grenade while in a helicopter. He was so close, he said, he could see the barrel of the rocket launcher. In reality, the helicopter that was attacked was half an hour ahead of his.

Similarly, Hillary Clinton once claimed she had been shot at by a sniper in a Bosnian airport, when in fact she had been warmly received there alongside the comedian Sinbad. Ronald Reagan once told a moving story of a World War II pilot who chose to go down with his gunner that later turned out to be the plot of a movie he had seen. It's safe to say the American public did not tolerate any of these blunders, viewing them all as outright lies. Most of the memory experts I spoke with, however, sympathized with these people, just as they'd sympathize with witnesses who thought they'd identified a criminal, only to find out years later they had remembered the wrong face,

When the Williams story broke, Loftus appeared in numerous media outlets, saying it was possible the man honestly believed his original story. This is not to imply that we should abandon our skepticism of public figures who stretch the truth, or that we shouldn't believe eyewitness testimony. But just as with other types of suggestion, none of us are immune to false memories. This, it seems, is who we are as humans—whether you're Hillary Clinton or someone who remembers being kidnapped by aliens or a confused kid wanting to please a grown-up.

An intelligent, creative person tells an emotionally rich story again and again, each time bringing up the memory, each time altering it just a little, thanks to the similarity of imagination and memory in the brain.[22] After a certain amount of retellings, the person honestly thinks the fabrication is reality. And whether it's Satan worshippers or aliens or snipers, the story is always more interesting and fantastic than the dingy truth. The truth is a man who paid for sex with kids in a poor neighborhood across town. The truth is a disorienting condition whereby you wake up and can't move while hallucinating little green men. The truth is a secretary of state disembarking her plane to attend another boring reception, shaking hands and smiling.

---

22 Among the first to lay out this proposition was a British team of researchers who wrote in 2003 that "thinking of the future is closely related to retrospective memory." They found that imagining the future and remembering the past use similar networks—kind of like how two roommates will frequent the same restaurants.

Some segments of law enforcement are becoming more aware that they may be unintentionally planting false memories. In 2014, the National Academies released an exhaustive review of the science behind tainted testimony and issued several recommendations, including videotaping the interview process and using double-blind police lineups, where neither the cops in the room nor the witness knows which person is the lead suspect (basically, the same way scientists avoid tipping off a subject that he might be getting a placebo pill).

There may not be much more we can do about filtering out false memories in the legal system. But imagine for a moment that we could somehow identify specific people susceptible to those kinds of memories. Let's say that *COMT* predicted a person's propensity to false memories (this work hasn't been done and there's little yet to suggest it would be true, but go with me). Suddenly, met/met testimony would be less valuable than val/val testimony. The courts currently operate on the notion that all people are equal under the law. But if you were on a jury and you knew that a person had a tendency toward false memories, would you trust him? Would we be relegating suggestible people to second-class citizenship?

The repercussions go even deeper. In 1938, a play called *Gas Light* hit the London stage and was turned into a popular movie six years later starring Ingrid Bergman and Charles Boyer. It's the story of a devious husband who, to make his wife think she's going crazy, tweaks certain elements of their home. One of the more effective techniques is to twiddle the gas knobs so that the lighting in the house grows dimmer and dimmer. All the while he adamantly denies anything is changing. "Gaslighting" has since referred to a surprisingly common phenomenon, especially in abusive relationships, whereby one person tries to make another doubt their own senses. Knowing that your own memories are not as reliable as your partner's would make you vulnerable to abuse.

It could also make you a target. Children and the mentally hand-icapped are victims of an unusually high number of assaults, partly because they make such terrible witnesses. What if sexual predators could target people prone to false memories? And several studies have suggested that women are more prone to memory errors than men are, providing an opportunity to discredit half the population. Is society ready for that kind of information?

That's the crucial difference between understanding individual variation in placebos versus in false memories. If we could somehow identify placebo-prone people, it would give doctors a whole suite of new and effective treatment options for them, while freeing up dozens or hundreds of new drugs for the rest of us. With false memories, however, the practical applications are frightening. Perhaps that's because our memories are so fundamental to who we are. Perhaps using expectation to manipulate thoughts is just more unsettling than using it to manipulate our bodies. If I close my eyes, I can see the side of Lost Arrow Spire I climbed 20 years ago during that lightning storm in Yosemite. I can see the wall, hear the roaring falls, and almost feel my heart clenching in my chest. But what if someone came to me tomorrow and told me it never happened? Or that it had happened to someone else? An emotionally charged, formative event that I've thought about hundreds of times since then is ripe for distortion.

When people ask me why I don't practice Christian Science any-more, I often point to that moment on that rock, 2,000 feet above the valley floor. Of course, my departure from my childhood religion was more complicated than that, but in the narrative I tell myself so that I can make sense of my own life, this was the moment when it all clicked.

What if that foundational memory isn't real? What does that make me? As with all forms of suggestion, false memories remind us that our perception of reality is fallible. Just as most of us are susceptible to placebos and some level of hypnosis, so too do we have to realize that *not everything we think happened actually did*. We are all vulnerable to suggestive storytelling that fits our own expectations. And if we are unable to see these memories as fallible, the consequences can be disastrous.

But that's not to say that false memories can't sometimes be helpful. In 2012, Loftus and a team at Yale, in collaboration with the U.S. Navy, did an experiment in which they interviewed soldiers who had endured tremendous hardship during a mock prisoner-of-war scenario. It's part of the Navy's attempt to prepare soldiers for the possible dangers of being captured behind enemy lines. Afterward, though, the team was easily able to alter details in the soldiers' memories: who their interrogator was, whether he had a weapon, whether there was a phone in the room.

What they found was that a person's memory was malleable right after a stressful situation—perhaps more malleable than usual. This corroborated a smaller study out of Yale a dozen years earlier, and raises tantalizing questions. What if false memories could be used to replace traumatic ones? What if they could be used to treat PTSD?

The U.S. Department of Veterans Affairs estimates that 10 percent of Afghanistan veterans, 20 percent of Iraq veterans, and a full 30 percent of Vietnam veterans experience some form of PTSD. What if there was a way to implant memories in a person that could dull the trauma of war? (Many hypnotherapists, going back to the 1880s, have acknowledged implanting false memories for therapeutic reasons.)

At the same time Loftus was working with the Navy, a team of MIT scientists targeted specific memories in specially designed mice. Using lasers, they actually added new memories to their minds (in this case, negative memories of a box that shocked their feet, though it could just as easily have been a positive memory). In essence, they gave the mice false memories. The experiment was a media sensation, amazing the world with the possibility of someday actually editing our experience of our past.

But for humans, this is a long way off—and obviously, going into a person's brain and changing a memory on purpose would carry huge ethical questions. But perhaps there might be a less drastic solution. Scientists in the laboratory have been able to change how the brain consolidates certain emotional memories using the drug propranolol. Essentially, it prevents the brain from filling the memory in correctly; eventually, it loses its destructive power. This process doesn't replace the memory per se. Instead, it applies the theory of false memory creation to take the edge off a little. We can boost the effect if the patient plays a video game or enters a virtual-reality world similar to the arena of memories that haunt the patient. But it's not clear that either of these solutions helps with long-term PTSD.

We often think of our mind, like our body, as a constant. Yes, we may injure our body on occasion or forget the name of our junior prom date, but we expect our mind and body to follow certain rules. Our body accurately reports to us what is happening, and when our mind tells us that something happened a certain way, that's the way it happened. But the science of suggestibility reveals this to be a fairy tale. In many cases, our body tells us just what our mind expects it to, and our mind remembers our life only in a way that fits our accepted narrative. And although it's true that being kidnapped by aliens or fed blood by satanists may seem like bizarre narratives, all one has to do is turn on the television to see that, in the modern world, we're frequently exposed to such stories. Strange as it may seem, for some of us, the notion that a creature traveled 13 light-years to collect our semen is easier to accept than the idea that our memories cannot be trusted.

But this is not the limit of suggestibility in our lives. Easing the pain of our body, the ruins of Parkinson's disease, and an upset stomach is impressive. Being able to conduct surgery on a conscious patient after just saying a few hypnotic words is even more so. And perhaps changing the very fabric of our memories is still more impressive. But suggestion is not limited to such momentous events; it's also quietly woven into the fabric of our daily lives. Exercise, eating, even sex—all are subject to the ever changing expectations of our chaotic, suggestible brain.

PART THREE

Suggestible Us

CHAPTER SEVEN

Sex, Drugs, *and* . . .

He is not deceived who knows himself
to be deceived.

—Latin legal maxim

A T THIS POINT, YOU MIGHT BE FORGIVEN for thinking that expectation and suggestion are limited to the realm of medicine. Certainly that's where they were discovered and that's where they play the most havoc. But they encompass so much more than that. Your ability to change *what is* into what you expect it to be can shape every facet of your day: what you buy and eat, how you exercise, and even what you look like and how you feel about yourself. Billions of dollars go into tinkering with, and then reinforcing, your expectations. Let's take a look at how this can play out in a few key areas of your life.

At the risk of sounding like a late-night infomercial, I can honestly say that suggestibility, if implemented correctly, has the power to make you thinner, happier, faster, stronger, smarter, more satisfied, and better in bed. Expectation can even make the food you eat taste better. And while it doesn't cost a cent, it does require that you buy something: the story being told.

While our brains are continually making predictions, there are also always stories around us that we can choose to believe—or not:

I knew it. She likes me. / *Nope. He hates me.*

This micro-beer is just as good as I heard it was. / *This cheap wine is awful.*

Damn, I look good—all those sit-ups must be working. / *I am a useless, stupid person, and no one will ever love me.*

These are all stories. And all of them, believe it or not, are subject to the whims of suggestion. If this seems shocking, believe me, it's nothing new to the people trying to capture our attention to sell us something every second of every day. For example, researchers have long known that food with a brand name tastes different from the exact same food put in a generic container. The same goes for two different brand names. Pepsi consistently pummels Coke in blind taste tests but is pummeled in return whenever tasters can see the labels. Similarly, wine that comes in an expensive-looking bottle with a lush description of its earthy tones, raspberry highlights, and slight hint of almond tastes better than the same wine in a plain bottle with no flowery words on the label. Notice that I didn't say, "it seems to taste better" or "we think it tastes better." According to psychologists, in all the ways that actually matter, it *does* taste better. It's not that gullible people eat cat food and think it's pâté; it's that they eat cat food and it becomes pâté.

OK, perhaps that's a bit of an exaggeration. Neuroscientists admit that if a bottle of wine is clearly bad—Welch's grape juice or nearly vinegar—people won't be duped into thinking it's a fine vintage. Expectation is an extraordinary force, but it can go only so far. No placebo is going to take away the pain of putting your hand in a pot of boiling water. No amount of suggestion will make you believe you used to be president of the United States. No amount of hypnosis can make you act against your values. And no fancy label is going to make you think grape juice is a 1945 Château Mouton Rothschild.

But when two products are roughly the same, expectation tends to play a far greater role in what we experience than do our senses. That's why, in a 2004 blind tasting, an unlabeled bottle of two-dollar Shiraz from Charles Shaw ("Two-Buck Chuck," as it's called at Trader Joe's) earned the Double Gold rating at the annual International Eastern Wine Competition, beating out thousands of other prestigious vintages. In 2007, its Chardonnay was named "Best in California" at the similarly competitive California Exposition and State Fair.

Psychologists have named this phenomenon a "marketing placebo," and over the past few years it has become all the rage. Just as with a pain placebo, it requires a healthy input from the reasoning, prefrontal parts of the brain.[23] Most companies achieve this in one of two ways: Either they spend a fortune creating, cultivating, and enhancing a particular brand, or they just use a good old-fashioned price tag. For example, if a company tells you it has a new line of brain-enhancing drinks—which, I shouldn't even have to tell you, is just flavored water—and you take a series of cognitive tests after imbibing, you'll find that your cognitive performance actually improves. If they tell you it's an especially expensive brand, your score will go up even more. That same principle applies to branding; studies suggest that athletes perform better when they drink flavored water out of a Gatorade bottle. And amazingly, students' test scores rise when they use a pen labeled "MIT."

As we have already learned, expensive placebos and placebos in name-brand bottles work better than cheap generics. And much of

---

23 In 2004, a Texas team tested this theory with the classic Pepsi versus Coke example—this time, inside a brain scanner. People first compared Pepsi and Coke without knowing which was which and then with the label exposed. In the first case, people preferred Pepsi and the pleasure centers deep within their brains lit up. But when the subjects knew what they were drinking, there was far more activity in the prefrontal cortex. And, of course, that time Coke won.

the research into marketing placebos mirrors the research on other types of suggestion. Marketing experts have even taken a stab at isolating the kinds of people and personalities that might best respond to suggestion (in the same way that others have tried to find the best responders to false memories, hypnosis, and placebos). The results seem to indicate that the people most suggestible to marketing are highly reward-seeking, are not particularly attuned to what their senses are telling them, and tend to really enjoy thinking (what psychologists call a "need for cognition"). The researchers who used the Gatorade bottle and the MIT pens correlated subjects' level of suggestibility to how they thought about the nature of intelligence and learning. Interestingly, those who thought of intelligence as more or less fixed—and thus perhaps intent on proving themselves—were more suggestible to brands than those who saw intelligence as more fluid. In other words, if you're the type of person who considers intelligence to be a malleable idea—that everyone has the capacity to be brilliant in their own way—then you may be less malleable to the power of marketing suggestions.

Of course, as with other types of suggestion, marketing placebos often require some form of deception, either from a caregiver or from oneself. From a cynical viewpoint, you might even say the history of commerce is one long chain of people trying to manipulate the suggestibility of their customers. In the end, as we've learned, the reach of expectation is not unlimited. You might be able to fool yourself into thinking that crappy pâté is delicious, though not that cat food is pâté. But what if there was a way to boost a marketing placebo?

Consider for a moment a $70 bottle of wine from a famous small family vineyard. Is it twice as good as a $35 bottle from another vineyard on the other side of town? Is it twice as expensive to make? Generally the answer is no (though good marketing ain't cheap). In fact, any economist will tell you that it's $70 because that's what people will pay for it. And if people will pay that much for it, well then it must be pretty good.

Does this logic sound familiar? It's a lot like Leonie Koban's experiment with placebos and peer pressure. She used marks on a screen inside an MRI that represented other people's reports of pain. In the case of good wine, expensive pâté, and a $50 cup of coffee, the price subconsciously reflects what others think it's worth. I wouldn't be surprised if someday we found out that drugs like vasopressin (which Luana Colloca used to boost the placebo effect) get released in your body when you have an expensive glass of wine. So next time you take a sip of a pricey wine, ask yourself whether it's expensive because of how good it tastes or whether it tastes so good because it's expensive.

● ● ●

Perhaps it's not so surprising that the way we experience food is subject to manipulation. Taste, after all, is subjective. Plus, dopamine plays a role in the desire to eat, and opioids likely play a role in our tastes. Eating is fundamentally a reward-driven activity, and lord knows we humans like our rewards. Sugar, fat, grease, candy—you name it. If someone wrapped a doughnut in bacon and dipped it in cake frosting, I would seriously consider eating it.

Which brings me to another part of our daily lives that scientists now say is all about suggestion. Namely, our ever expanding waistlines. In the same way that our instinctual fears, which protected our ancestors for millions of years, can get out of control and create nocebos that affect our bodies, so, too, can our ancient need for sweet and fattening food get us in trouble in the modern world.

A 2015 Finnish study showed that obesity is tied to the number of opioid receptors in the brain (drug addicts, as we will see, often have a similar problem, except with dopamine receptors).[24] In other words, with fewer opportunities for pleasure-related endorphins, some people seek out more pleasurable experiences like eating. It's not that addiction and overeating are the same thing; it's just that they manifest in very similar ways.

That's how the calories get into our body. But what about how our body reacts to them? Does expectation play a role in gaining and losing weight? If expectation can make you well, make you sick, ease your pain, and even kill you, then it's a good bet that it can trim down that spare tire too. Scientists have discovered a fascinating web of interconnected chemicals that link your brain and your belly, many of which may harness placebo-like effects when you start that new fad diet or that all-fruit purge.

Actually, fad diets and alternative healing methods have a lot in common and often overlap quite a bit, since things like fruit diets and vitamin infusions promise to make you both healthy and thin. Then there's the antioxidant craze that claims to make you healthier by attacking the evil "free radicals" in your body. Free radicals—extra ions floating in your bloodstream—are in some ways as natural as pomegranate juice and are an important part of your body's functioning. It's true that if they get too plentiful, they can lead to cancer, but the same would be true if they got too scarce. And it's certainly not clear that drinking smoothies can somehow eradicate free radicals and protect you from cancer.

This same expectation game applies to "toxins." Fat-soluble pollutants can't leave our bodies except through breastfeeding, and our kidneys don't need any help getting rid of water-soluble ones. Any diet or form of exercise that claims to make you healthy by purging

---

24 Interestingly, the number of dopamine receptors is the same for both groups. But for some reason, obesity seems tied more to opioid receptors whereas addiction seems more tied to dopamine.

toxins is just playing with your suggestibility. Evil free radicals and toxins are just stories. We buy them or we don't.

The same may be true for the Atkins diet, the all-cabbage diet, the morning-banana diet, the werewolf diet, and the Hollywood cookie diet, as well as the Israeli army diet, the Master Cleanse, the Zone diet, macrobiotics, the alkaline diet, and the baby-food diet (yes, these are all real). Of course, all of these regimens contain a few shreds of science, some of which might be completely valid. But they also involve elaborate storytelling that sounds a lot like the placebo paradigms we've seen before.

My favorite example of creative health storytelling is green coffee bean extract, which is basically a supplement made from unroasted coffee beans. For years, every huckster and health charlatan on late-night and daytime TV claimed it was a miracle diet pill and even a cancer treatment—despite the fact that it's essentially the same thing millions of Americans already drink every day. The miracle claims were based on the presence of something called chlorogenic acid, which largely burns off when coffee beans are roasted. One study out of the University of Scranton claimed that thanks to this wondrous chemical, 16 overweight people lost an average of almost 18 pounds and 16 percent of their body fat over a six-week period. Just from taking green coffee bean extract and exercising. Which is incredible. So incredible that it's not true.

You see, the study wasn't done in Scranton; it was done in India and funded by a company called Applied Food Sciences that sold the supplement. According to the Federal Trade Commission (which eventually fined the company $3.5 million), the study was so overwhelmingly botched, with data altered and changes made to the parameters halfway through, that they couldn't publish it. So the company pawned it off on someone else to publish—academics at a small school who, according to the Federal Trade Commission, noticed a few irregularities but never asked any questions. The final paper (which was retracted) mentioned the company as having only donated the pills used in the experiment, not that it actually conducted the experiment.[25]

In the end, it probably isn't the chlorogenic acid in the green coffee bean extract that helps people lose weight; it's plain old caffeine. After all, caffeine is a mild performance-enhancing drug and may help slightly with weight loss. But even the caffeine pales before the most powerful ingredient: a healthy dose of suggestion. To better understand how suggestion affects our waistlines, I called Alia Crum, a young, upcoming psychology researcher at Stanford University.

For the past decade, Crum has been looking at all sorts of ways that expectation affects people's lives. But instead of focusing just on placebos or expectations, she widens her research out to what she calls "mindsets," a shorthand for the many vagaries that separate one human mind from the next. In 2010, she conducted an experiment with milkshakes, comparing the effects of a 140-calorie diet shake (which came with a sensible, diet-shake label) with those of a 620-calorie shake (carrying a delicious-sounding, indulgent label). That's roughly the same as eating a small salad versus a double-patty cheeseburger with all the fixings. Except that, of course, she was lying. Both shakes were really about 380 calories.

Crum tracked the amount of ghrelin produced in the bodies of her subjects. Ghrelin is a fascinating little hormone that our stomach secretes to tell us we are hungry. It also seems to play a role in monitoring how energy is absorbed in the body. But notice that all these

---

25 But that didn't stop health gurus from picking it up. The most notable was Dr. Oz, who called it a "miracle pill." It's not the first time he's held up snake oil as medicine (a Canadian study showed that fewer than half his recommendations are backed up, and 14 percent are actually contradicted, by science), but it did force him to admit to Congress that on his show, he's an entertainer, not a doctor.

things start in the body, not the mind. The stomach tells the brain when it's hungry, not the other way around. Ghrelin tapers off after we eat and we are no longer hungry because the stomach is full. But Crum found that sometimes the process can work in reverse. When she told subjects she was giving them a fattening shake, their ghrelin levels were far lower than those of the people who thought they were getting a diet shake. Remember, everyone got the *same* shake—the only difference was expectation.[26]

In other words, their brains were telling their stomachs how to do their jobs. It's a little like an intra-body Jedi mind trick. The stomach calls the brain and says, "I'm empty. You're hungry." And the brain calls back down and says, "I'm full and so are you." And in a flat tone of voice, the stomach responds, "Yes. You are full and so am I."

So what can we make of this? Well, we can guess that weight loss, like so many other conditions in the body, is subject to the whims of expectation. Of course we can't really say how much because few of these experiments are properly controlled and almost none of the diets are rigorously tested (for which you would need to devise some kind of placebo salad). Also, in many cases, including the botched green coffee bean extract study, the subjects are required to exercise, which itself might be driving the weight loss. Still, it's clear that it's impossible to separate the role of a diet from the role of your expectation of that diet.

Or maybe you don't even need a diet. Maybe a little perspective is enough to give you a healthier lifestyle. "It's not just what you're doing; it's how you're thinking about what you're doing," Crum says.

---

26 Ghrelin, discovered in 1999, is a relatively new hormonal player, and scientists are still working out how it functions. But along with its sister, leptin (which tells the brain "I'm full"), it's linked to conditions like obesity and anorexia. They are also tied to the nocebo chemical CCK. It turns out that it's CCK's job to shut down ghrelin when the stomach is full.

"And what sort of mindsets or expectations you have that encapsulate those things."

As it happens, Crum has her own connection to Christian Science. Her mother was raised in the religion, and her grandmother was a professional healer. And although neither she nor her mother practices anymore, Christian Science has deeply affected their outlook on life and Crum's approach to her work. Her mother constantly encouraged her daughter to alter her mindset whenever she was sick. "When she went through menopause, she told me that she decided to view those hot flashes as cutting calories," she says.

As an undergraduate at Harvard, Crum was an acolyte of the legendary firebrand psychologist Ellen Langer. Decades before, Langer had conducted a famous experiment in which elderly people felt younger when immersed in the trappings of their younger days. In 2006, Crum recruited 84 hotel chambermaids to participate in a simple experiment to see whether she could similarly improve people's health—not by tricking them, but by telling them the truth. She started out by conducting interviews with the maids who spend their days on their feet, walking from room to room, pushing vacuums, and doing a hundred other straightforward physical tasks. She took their blood pressure, weight, and a number of other health indicators. Then she asked them how much exercise they got per week. Most of them said not a lot.

Next, she took half the maids and gave them a short tutorial that explained the value of their work as exercise, citing that they actually got well more daily activity than the surgeon general recommends. A month later, she revisited both groups; those who had received the tutorial experienced a significant weight loss and drop in blood pressure when compared with their co-workers. They also had more energy after work and a new outlook on the work they did.

The study wasn't long enough to track weight loss over time, though Crum has always been curious to see just how far belief can take a person's health. We can't expect to see our pounds magically float away because we believe they will. But then again, we still don't know just how far our beliefs will go in determining how healthy we feel.

"I don't think the power of mind is limitless," Crum says. "But I do think we don't yet know where those limits are."

For an even better look at the role of expectation on fitness, we can go to the other extreme and consider competitive athletes. Everyone knows that athletes are superstitious—wearing gold thongs under their uniforms or refusing to change their socks—and are thus susceptible to certain . . . let's call them performance nocebos. But what about the body's ability to perform? Can you supercharge your muscles purely by suggestion? You bet your gold jockstrap you can.

Back in the 1970s, scientists at the University of Massachusetts Amherst selected 6 varsity athletes from a group of 15, ostensibly to test how much better they would perform than their cohorts while using anabolic steroids. So they pulled them into a room and extolled the virtues of juicing. Once the athletes were sufficiently pumped up to get pumped up, they started a seven-week period of heavy weight-lifting (including bench presses, military presses, and squats), with no drugs. Then, for another four weeks they were given steroids that were actually placebo pills. As you might expect, the six pseudo-dopers increased in strength, not only beyond that of their fellow students who hadn't been fed the stories and pills but also beyond their own performance during the initial workout period.

At the time, this finding brought up more questions than it did answers. What's the mechanism? Is the body mimicking steroid release? (And, by the way, did anyone ever tell the kids at the end that it was all fake and that drugs are bad?) Since then, numerous studies have administered placebos to athletes in the guise of performance-enhancing drugs. One 2015 study experimented with runners who thought they were blood doping—the illegal technique of adding red blood cells to your body made famous by cyclist Lance Armstrong's colossal fall from grace. Of course, the runners weren't getting infused with blood but with simple saltwater; yet they still shaved 1.2 percent from their times (which is a lot for runners, who are thrilled to shave off even a few seconds). A 2008 study demonstrated that weightlifters improved their performance by 12 percent to 16 percent when they thought they were taking caffeine (a known, albeit legal, performance enhancer) but were actually only taking placebos. Then the experimenters went a step further with a second group by adding a layer: They reduced the amount of weight being lifted without telling the subjects, making them believe that they were getting stronger on the placebo. The easier experience confirmed the participants' expectation about the pills and nearly doubled the amount of actual weight they could lift. Similar studies have played with fake steroids, supplements, oxygenated water, amino acids, and even sodium bicarbonate, which goes by the street name "baking soda."[27]

Fabrizio Benedetti, whom you may remember as pioneering some of the most telling nocebo studies of the 1990s, has also conducted hundreds of placebo studies, including a fascinating one using morphine. His subjects simulated a workout by doing special arm exercises designed to measure how well people tolerate pain. It burns like a workout because your arms are deprived of oxygen. The logic is that all painkillers are performance enhancers (*no pain, no gain*, right?). Sure enough, the subjects doing the exercise with no promise of performance enhancement became about 7.5 percent more resistant to the pain of the workout, just through practice. If they were told they were getting morphine to enhance their performance but received a

---

27 Believe it or not, baking soda is a moderate performance enhancer. Acidosis, or the overabundance of H+ ions in the body, is a key part of exhaustion, and apparently ingesting baking soda helps the spaces between cells resist the effects of acidosis. It has not yet been banned by the Olympics.

placebo, they became 18 percent better. And if they actually received morphine for a while and then switched to a placebo, they became *50 percent* more resistant to the exercise pain. But if they got the placebo-killing drug naloxone, all the gains vanished.

So how are these people increasing their performance? Although these are not professional athletes, they are serious about their sports, and even a 12 percent enhancement is tough to explain, let alone 50 percent. It could be that there is a not-yet-understood mechanism at work that is actually building strength-boosting red blood cells. Or it could be that it's our own natural opioids. Perhaps without the pain of the taxed muscles, it's possible to outperform your best expectations. In that case, I suppose the saying should be *no pain, more gain.*

But this also brings up an interesting question. It's illegal to use drugs like morphine in the Olympics—not only because it's unsafe to cover up potentially serious injuries but also because that loss of pain creates an unfairly enhanced performance. But what if someone were to use morphine only while training and then use placebos during the match? That's not technically cheating, and there wouldn't be traces of it by the day of the match. By then, the athlete's own brain would be providing the illegal performance-enhancing drugs. Can our own opioids be illegal substances? Take it one step further: Forget about cheating altogether. Looking at two clean athletes, how can we be sure that the difference between a 4-minute mile and a 3-minute-and-59-second mile isn't just a slightly better internal pharmacy? It kind of changes the meaning of the phrase "level playing field."

Baseball savant Yogi Berra once said, "Baseball is ninety percent mental. The other half is physical." At the time, people just made fun of his math skills. But with our growing understanding of the power of the brain to enhance everything from cycling to tennis to weightlifting, it's starting to look as if Yogi was correct. Sports are 100 percent mental and physical—and maybe 50 percent suggestion.

• • •

Looking thinner, running faster, and enjoying your food are wonderful perks of expectation. But the science of expectation reaches far deeper into our lives than that. The same themes that drive expectation and rewards can send some people into a dark, hellish place. And sometimes bring them back again.

The most obvious of these themes is addiction. Approximately 1 in 10 Americans is addicted to some kind of drug—mostly alcohol. Addiction was once viewed as a moral failing or a lack of willpower, but today we understand it as mostly physiological, specifically around our old friend dopamine (which isn't surprising, since the neurotransmitter deals with anticipation and enjoyment of rewards). That can mean sugar, sex, money, a high score on Grand Theft Auto—or using drugs.

But drug use doesn't just change the way you feel for a couple of hours; it can also change the brain itself. When presented with an abundance of pleasurable chemical stimulation through drug use, the nervous system will get overwhelmed and shut down its production of dopamine to bring itself back into equilibrium. In a bad feedback loop, the person then finds himself short on dopamine whenever he's not using the drug. Food doesn't taste as good, and even sex loses its thrill. The only way to get back to normal is to take the drug that caused the problem in the first place.

But it's more than that. Some scientists say addiction literally changes the way the brain works. Not only do addicts have less dopamine from drug overuse, but also their dopamine receptors are affected (either changing their numbers or changing how well they transmit messages). Additionally, regular drug use actually twists our memories so that we crave both the drug and the circumstances surrounding the drug use (which is why people crave a cigarette and also pulling it from the pack and lighting it). Meanwhile, addiction causes the brain's impulse control centers to shut down, guaranteeing relapse. Remember how Karin Jensen trained people's brains to release a placebo response when they saw an image of a face flicker so quickly they couldn't consciously register it? The same thing happens with cocaine addicts. Show them an image of blow for just 33 milliseconds—too fast for the conscious brain to take in—and they will have immediate cravings.

Almost all the world's favorite recreational drugs either mimic or employ chemicals similar to the ones we tap into with expectation. In fact, the more I learn about addiction, the more I see it as a sort of perversion of all the brain circuits and processes explored in this book. By the same token, suggestion and expectation may hold the answers to overcoming it. Naloxone—the drug that first helped expose the chemical nature of placebos and that blocks placebo responses altogether—wasn't invented for placebo research. Today, it serves a crucial role in medicine as an emergency treatment for drug overdoses. Just as it blocks the effects of our internal pharmacy, it's also pretty effective at blocking the effects of, say, heroin or oxycodone. And a closely related drug, naltrexone, is one of the most effective ways to treat alcohol abuse.

Hard to believe? Next time your favorite drinking buddy comes over, serve him a nonalcoholic beer in a bottle for alcoholic beer. Make it three. Can you guess what happens next? Multiple studies have shown that people who think they're drinking booze but are actually drinking a nonalcoholic brew feel just as drunk as those drinking the real stuff—at least for a couple drinks. Mind you, their blood alcohol levels are still zero, but they feel tipsy. And you can also go the other way: Give someone alcohol but tell her it's root beer. One study out of Minot State University in North Dakota doctored a root beer to give it the same alcohol level as beer. The researchers offered the doctored drink to a group of unsuspecting volunteers while another group received regular beer. Presumably, both groups got tipsy after a few drinks, but that wasn't the point. Those who drank beer actually absorbed more alcohol into their blood than those who thought they were drinking soda but were in fact consuming just as much alcohol—almost as if the beer drinkers' bodies were absorbing booze partly because they expected to. (To be fair, part of this reaction might be due to the way alcohol is absorbed with malt from beer versus sugar from soda.)

But changing our expectation can have an even more profound impact on addiction. One of its most insidious forms is to prescription drugs. Here is a medicine specifically tailored to relieve a patient's suffering that winds up causing a whole new type of suffering. Some two million Americans are addicted to prescription opioid drugs, and about 19,000 died from overdoses in 2014 alone. For perspective, that's about twice the number who died from heroin overdoses, and three times the number who died from cocaine.

There may be a very good reason for this. One theory of pain holds that after an injury, the pain never leaves; it just gets gradually covered up by the body's internal medicine cabinet—like a lamp that slowly gets dimmer as the sun comes up. A team out of the University of Kentucky decided to test this in 2013. Led by Bradley Taylor (a student of Howard Fields, the scientist who first discovered the chemical nature of placebos back in the 1970s), the team gave naloxone to patients who had recovered from an injury and, sure enough, for many of them the pain came right back. Presumably because it had been there the whole time, hiding under the surface.

Even more surprising, the patients displayed some of the hallmarks of opioid withdrawal. That's right: During the process of recovering from pain, we actually become dependent on our own opioids. This,

Taylor thinks, may be the key to understanding not only addiction but also the switch from short-term to chronic pain.

Still, being dependent on your own internal drugs is far better than being dependent on prescription drugs. So what would happen if rather than replacing your own natural pain relievers with drugs, we just administered the natural stuff? NIH researcher Luana Colloca is trying to do just that. In 2016 she began a project that blends the best of placebo research and pain relief to try to beat addiction before it starts. To achieve this, she mixed a few placebo pills into a group of pain patients' medication. Each week they might have five or six pain pills and one or two placebos. As the month progressed, she upped the placebos and dropped the opioids until the artificial drug was administered only about half the time.

Do you see what's happening? First she trains the patient to expect pain relief when taking a pill. Then she takes the pill away and lets the patient's own expectation cover the pain relief, just as she did with me in that electrocution chair. Rather than becoming dependent on the drug, which would lessen the effect of the internal pharmacy, the patient uses her expectation to switch from an external drug to an internal one. If addiction is the corruption of everything that's good about expectation, why not use expectation to smother addiction before it has a chance to begin?

● ● ●

Addiction is not the only way that brain chemistry can wreak havoc on your life. There is another condition just as insidious, just as stigmatized, and just as vulnerable to suggestion: depression.

I felt depressed at 18 when I didn't get into my first-choice college. And again when I left a career in biology, and again last year when I ripped a tendon in my ankle and had to have surgery. I was bummed out and slept too much and wasn't fun to be around. But although I might think that these experiences inform me about depression, they don't.

Clinical depression is not the same as being bummed out because your favorite college rejected you. It's a physiological disease that alters your brain functioning in a measurable way, can ruin your life, and can even kill you. Depression isn't a sadder version of you; it's a whole different you. The best way to describe it is like being chemically sedated into someone you don't recognize. Because, in a way, you are. I've never been clinically depressed, but I know enough about brain chemistry to say that, given the choice, I might prefer excruciating chronic pain. Not that patients get that choice; for many, clinical depression and chronic pain go hand in hand. And the numbers for depression, like chronic pain, are staggering. Some 7 percent of Americans will experience clinical depression this year, costing the United States more than $200 billion.

Scientists going back to the early 2000s have found that just as depression has tangible effects on the brain, so does expectation, but in reverse. In fact, placebos and expectation are so effective against depression that it is difficult to find a drug that's more powerful. From 1987 to 1999 the pharmaceutical industry exploded with depression meds like Prozac, Paxil, Zoloft, Luvox, and Celexa—each of which has become a blockbuster drug and presumably helped millions of suffering people. But if you look at drug studies during this time, about 75 to 80 percent of their efficacy can be attributed to placebo effects. And if you look carefully, there was no real difference between high doses and low doses, which is odd and suggests the meds weren't as effective as we thought. (Usually, for a truly effective drug, you would expect a difference. Imagine a high dose of morphine versus a small one.)

What's more, these effects seem to be long-lived—for weeks and months even. It didn't do any good to exclude placebo responders in the first few weeks; others just filled their place. This high placebo response has been one of the main reasons why depression has been so difficult and expensive to treat. Just as with painkillers, depression drugs have a massive, unscalable impediment between research and FDA certification. Not that people haven't tried. Prozac first hit the market in 1988, after it barely outperformed the placebo. More recently it looked like deep-brain stimulation—electronic devices implanted into the brain to stimulate a specific region directly—might become a breakthrough technology capable of eradicating serious depression once and for all. But over the past few years, that, too, has come under serious criticism and seems unable to beat the placebo effect.[28]

It could be that deep brain stimulation either isn't ready for clinical use or never had the potential that researchers hoped it did. But there's another, perhaps more vexing possibility. Over the past few decades, scientists have noticed a distinct uptick in the power of the placebo effect on pain and depression trials. As discussed earlier, some experts even say that if Prozac had to compete against the placebo effect today, it would not have been cleared by the FDA. (Remember that once a drug clears the Phase III, placebo-controlled trial, it is certified—regardless of how it performs in later experiments.)

What happened? The drugs haven't gotten weaker, and it's not likely that people can build up an immunity to Prozac-like drugs. No, it seems that over time, the placebo effect itself has gotten stronger. How is that possible? Well, depressed patients not already taking an antidepressant are increasingly hard to find in the United States. So many companies are going offshore, where there are different cultural norms and where perhaps Western doctors might be more impressive and boost expectations. But an easier explanation would be that our own

---

28 It's possible that there is a difference in placebo response between major depression and mild depression. Some scientists say that people with mild depression are more placebo prone and thus skew the results.

expectation of what a depression drug can do has changed. Back in the mid-1980s no one knew what Prozac was or what to expect. But today, everyone knows of the Prozac brand, and people come to it with plenty of preconceived notions about what it's going to do. Perhaps Prozac beat the medical placebo only to be bulldozed by a marketing one.

If it's true that placebo rates are rising across the board, it's not clear what we can do about it. Perhaps rather than fighting expectation, we could embrace it. As with depression drugs, sleeping pills are facing a similar placebo crisis. One 2005 NIH study showed that although sleeping pills are effective, they provide only an average of 10 extra minutes of sleep per night when compared with sugar pills. But rather than fight expectation, some experts are embracing it. So why fight it? A 2015 study out of the University of Pennsylvania found that one of the best ways to get a good night's sleep is to mix your jar of sleeping pills with placebos, so that on a given night you wouldn't know which you were taking.

• • •

Not all drugs have the problems of Prozac or Ambien. Occasionally, one comes along that is so obviously effective that it obliterates the need for brain-based treatments. For this, we turn our attention to the ultimate form of reward processing—more gratifying than food, exercise, and probably even drugs. And that's sex.

Sexual placebos are probably older than any other form of suggestibility on Earth. For thousands of years, humans have used a long and diverse list of ingredients to treat sexual dysfunction in men and enhance sexual pleasure in women. If you want to better your skills between the sheets, according to a wide variety of cultures, you can try ginseng, powdered tiger penis, an African conifer called yohimbe, duck embryo boiled alive, the bark of the Mediterranean cluster pine,[29] the brain of a live monkey, horny goat weed, sea cucumber, dog meat, and, of course, oysters.

It almost goes without saying that dopamine and sex are strongly linked. After all, what's more rewarding—evolutionarily, biologically, or personally—than sex? Obviously, expectation plays an enormous role in its physiological buildup and enjoyment. Scientists have studied how dopamine can crash in lovers who stay together long periods of time without maintaining their relationship.[30] And for hundreds of years, the only way to enhance your sexual prowess was through various types of suggestion. But for men, that all changed with UK92480.

In the early 1990s, scientists at the drug company Pfizer were working on a failed heart medication they called UK92480 when they noticed an odd side effect. The men who used it reported raging erections several days after taking the medication. Rather than write this off as a humorous anecdote, the researchers changed the whole drug strategy. Thus was born sildenafil citrate, more commonly known as Viagra. It hit the market in 1997, and almost overnight erectile dysfunction was cured in all but the most serious cases. Never before had an entire class of ancient herbal and alternative treatments become so obsolete so quickly. Why spend $1,300 for tiger penis or $100 for a gram of caterpillar fungus when you can be guaranteed an erection for less than $2?

Viagra also created a lot of interesting opportunities to study placebos in erectile dysfunction. Early studies showed that a little more

---

29 *Pinus pinaster*—the name alone inspires confidence.

30 Generally, "maintaining" means lots of affectionate and sexual touching. Without that, the dopamine spike tends to drop over time as part of something called the Coolidge effect. The best way to bring it up to its original level is to bring in a new mate (the effect exists in both sexes but is stronger in men). The effect is named for President Calvin Coolidge, whose wife supposedly once noted to him how much sex roosters have. He responded that a rooster has more than one hen to choose from.

than half the time, Viagra-like drugs immediately helped sexually dysfunctional men have intercourse. With just a little persistence and patience, more than 80 percent of them eventually had success. Perhaps not surprisingly, the placebo group fared worse, though not as badly as you would expect. The placebo group had about a 20 percent success rate as soon as they popped the pill and about 50 percent if they persisted. Even men with erectile dysfunction resulting from spinal injury have been able to have sex after taking a placebo.

Conversely, one study revealed that if you tell someone that the drug he's taking will cause erectile dysfunction, loss of libido, or ejaculation problems, he's three times as likely to experience one of those problems as a man taking the same drug who was not given one of those assessments. Call it a sex nocebo.

Research has shown that expectation plays a role in women's sexual dysfunction as well—although, par for the course, there are far fewer studies. One very small experiment suggested that women with arousal and orgasmic dysfunctions improved on placebos over eight weeks, especially if they were older and had been with their partner longer. For years, scientists have been searching for a female Viagra, especially something that could be marketed to women postmenopause. Several such drugs have proved very effective but were stymied—not by high placebo responses, but by negative side effects such as loss of energy, dizziness, and nausea. Finally, in August 2015, the FDA approved a drug called Addyi, which was only about 10 percent more effective than a placebo and requires users to abstain from alcohol while using it. So far it hasn't been terribly popular.

Meanwhile, plenty of placebos throughout the years have helped women battling infertility. Women hoping to become mothers have tried vaginal steam baths, moonstone, rubbing a pregnant woman's belly, rubbing a statue's belly, tying a hen to the bedpost on their wedding night, wearing orange panties, eating lotus flowers, sacrificing a rabbit, and—perhaps the creepiest therapy—rocking an empty cradle. In Ireland, young couples were once encouraged to drink lots of honey wine (which, come to think of it, is basically the same thing many couples do today).

Perhaps some historical fertility cures—rosemary, parsley, and hazelnut—do indeed have some as-yet-undiscovered mechanism, some pharmacological value. Perhaps it's just a numbers game. The more time that goes by while a couple tries various remedies, the more likely that they will get pregnant. Or perhaps there is something more. Plenty of experts have suggested there might be a connection between stress and infertility, and most doctors will tell you to avoid stress if you're struggling to conceive. Not much evidence has surfaced, but in 2014 one team at Ohio State University found that out of 500 couples, the most stressed-out women were about 30 percent more likely to have problems conceiving. Other studies show that when a couple doesn't conceive, men are more likely to have erectile dysfunction. And back and forth it goes.

In the end, when it comes to human reproduction and expectation, erectile dysfunction and Viagra still offer the clearest glimpse into how our brains tug the strings in our bodies. Viagra has also offered a unique opportunity to observe what happens when thousands of years of suggestibility collide with a highly effective drug. Erectile dysfunction has been one of the most popular targets in history for alternative remedies. With the availability of Viagra, shouldn't monkey brain and horny goat weed disappear from the market? Unfortunately—especially when it comes to aphrodisiacs that come from endangered animals—the answer is no. Instead, Viagra started popping up in alternative products across the board. According to one 2009 FDA estimate, more than a third of sexual-enhancement supplements contain the active ingredient in Viagra, sometimes at twice the normal dose. Among them are supposedly natural products with names like

Vigor-25, Lady Shanghai, True Man, Strong Testis, and, apparently without irony, Blue Steel.

The inclusion of Viagra in herbal supplements illustrates the delicate balance that our beliefs play in the modern world. For centuries, there wasn't much modern medicine could offer those who suffered from erectile dysfunction. Harnessing expectation instead worked reasonably well. Then Viagra appeared. Overnight, there was an option that clearly surpassed any form of suggestion or miracle herbal cure. Suggestibility, it seems, has its limits.

As someone who was raised using nothing but my belief to treat my body, I have a deep-seated respect for the power of expectation. But as someone who was also raised to fear aspirin, I remember the first time I tried it and felt my headache disappear. Belief is an amazing and mysterious thing, but there is nothing quite as impressive as a drug that really works. And when faced with the, uh, towering success of Viagra, belief-based cures had no choice but to either surpass it or become obsolete. It's not the branding or belief alone that allows Viagra to work. It's the effective medicine in that pill.

● ● ●

We can see how placebo logic plays a significant role in how we experience flavors, weight loss, addictions, depression, and sex, among many other things. But I can't help wondering how much of a role memory plays in supercharging expectation. When you try that fad diet and you start to see results, for whatever reason, those results increase your sense of expectation ("Hey, this is working!"). But a year later, when you think back on that time, how accurate is your memory? Judging from the work of false-memory researchers, it would seem that your memory of that moment would become ever more dramatic ("Within days, I had shed all that weight!"). What about that $500 bottle of 1972 wine you shared with your rich uncle Norbert 10 years ago? Certainly the wine had gotten better with age, but hasn't your memory too?

The same forces are at play with other placebos. *As soon as I took the pill, the pain was gone! The moment the shaman touched me, I was healed!* Having seen and heard about many healings as a boy, I noticed that the stories became more dramatic as time went on. Recoveries became instant recoveries. A doctor with a frank diagnosis became a doctor who had given up all hope. A particularly low point in the disease became a deathbed. Healing became a miracle. How often this happens, I cannot say. But any memory charged with a lot of emotion that is revisited again and again is subject to distortion—and that distortion is likely to fit a narrative that increases your expectation for the next time. Suddenly, you remember those herbs you took as the defining moment in your cure. That acupuncture session made the pain dissolve instantly.

We know from other placebo studies that reinforced expectation only becomes stronger, and so the next time, your expectation for that diet, that wine, or that shaman is even higher: the classical conditioning of memory, if you will. How many people's amazing recoveries from sickness actually happened the way they think they did? And do we care—so long as they worked?

Expectation is suffused into every facet of our daily lives. It's likely a foundational part of our evolution. Today, its triggers can be seen on every billboard and every toothpaste commercial, attached to almost every product you can imagine. Is it any wonder that our minds are getting ahead of our bodies? When should you embrace your suggestibility and when should you be wary of it?

In the beginning of the book, I listed a few medieval concoctions that people used to believe could make them well. The point was to show how suggestibility can change with the fashion of the times and maybe make you laugh a little at the ridiculousness of those remedies. But I went online the other day and read about some of the latest trends in beauty treatments. There were skin treatments made from snail slime, bird poop, urine, bee venom, and placenta and—I had trouble believing this one—human blood facials. When it comes to heart surgery, antibiotics, and erections, modern medicine has changed the game. When it comes to vanity, though, it seems not much has changed.

There's a surprising amount you can do to harness the power of expectation and suggestion in your own life. If the poorest man on Earth honestly sees himself as a king, is he not a king? And if the wealthiest man among us sees himself as a miserable wretch, what is he but a miserable wretch? And if either man were to change what he is, the first thing that would have to change would be his own perception. The whirligig of emotions and beliefs and memories that make up our consciousness is one of nature's greatest creations. Minds just like ours have moved mountains, built wonders, and composed works of genius. In every case, those people were ruled not by what was but by what they expected. And occasionally, what they expected was possible. Your mind is the greatest prediction machine the world has ever known. Where you decide to place those expectations is up to you.

CHAPTER EIGHT

Harnessing *the* Power *of* Expectation

*Let us pretend in order to make the pretence
into a reality.*

—C. S. Lewis

W E ARE, ALL OF US, SUGGESTIBLE. There is no escaping our gullible brains. Not all our expectations are going to be true. When they're not, the mistakes show up in our bodies. I can't tell you how many times in the course of writing this book I heard someone say, "I'm not someone who believes in this stuff, but [fill in the blank] really works!" Whether it's Saint-John's-wort or ginseng or the light of the new moon on bare skin, if it works, then yes, you are someone who believes in this stuff. We all are. Some of that belief is subconscious, and some of it is just a response to damn good storytelling. But none of us can say there isn't something out there—some perfectly framed suggestion—that won't make us sick or make us well.

Think about your heart. Certainly there is no more mechanistic organ in your body—impervious to placebos and psychology, right? It's a muscled pump that does its job every second of every day; if you want to replace it, you can literally put a machine in its stead. And yet prolonged fear, anxiety, and stress can stop it mid-beat. Furthermore, numerous studies have shown the heart is just as placebo prone as any other organ in your body. Beta-blockers have failed, thanks to high placebo responses, as have pacemakers.

All of the studies using placebos to treat heart conditions have focused on non-lethal heart problems like arrhythmias and sudden lightheadedness. Interestingly, just as Parkinson's surgeries are more potent than sham Parkinson's drugs, sham pacemakers are more effective than sham heart medication. It's possible that these same effects play a role in more lethal heart conditions, but those kinds of experiments would require people with life-threatening illness to get a placebo. And although this certainly happens, it shouldn't in the halls of science.

But it's not really surprising that this pump in your chest might respond to your thoughts and expectations. After all, no cardiologist on Earth would argue that if you want to cure your heart, you need to address not just its mechanics but also your diet, lifestyle, and emotional life. So why is it any different for pain, influenza, or a broken leg?

The body's ability to heal itself through expectation and self-deception has been evident for tens of thousands, hundreds of thousands, maybe millions of years. It's built into who we are. Three thousand years ago, people gathered in sacred spaces to chant themselves into a hypnotic state. They rubbed dung on open wounds and mixed potent herbs with inert ones, hoping that one of them would cure their diseases. They told stories that became ever more improbable. It's pointless to pretend we are somehow impervious to suggestion's power.

Earlier I asked how you can treat a disease if you don't know whether it's real. Perhaps that is the wrong question. Perhaps we should stop acting as if there is some kind of line between the mind and the body. In the same way that placebos can be as powerful as drugs or a few hypnotic words can erase real pain, any disease that cripples a person, whether it begins in the body or the mind, is absolutely real.

So how can we use this knowledge in our daily lives? To harness the power of expectation, first you have to understand that any placebo or hypnotic induction is nothing more than a device for storytelling. It's an expectation vessel that works only if it can capture your imagination. So what kinds of stories engage you? What source of authority inspires the most confidence in you? Scientists and engineers? Ancient wisdom? Are you someone who craves quiet solitude or a social person who loves the teeming masses soaked in vasopressin?

The first thing University of Washington researcher David Patterson did when he tried to hypnotize me was get to know my personal history. He asked me about my father and his arm troubles after playing professional baseball. It wasn't that he thought my dad's arm pain was connected to mine; he just needed a story that resonated with me and thus tapped into my belief and expectation.

But wait, you might say: If I start thinking about health care as storytelling, doesn't that rob the story of its power? Like the magician who drops the hidden card from his sleeve? For some people this may be true. But remember that much of the power of suggestion happens outside our conscious awareness. Karin Jensen, the Harvard researcher who used faces to cue placebos, was able to demonstrate that many placebos happen subconsciously. Her colleague Ted Kaptchuk showed that a placebo can work even when you know it's a placebo. In that way, the placebo effect may be more like hypnosis than we realize; it just requires your willingness to be open. When you go to a magic show, do you believe the woman is actually sawed in half? No. You go to witness the illusion—the spectacle—and to let it fool you as much as your brain will allow. But if the magician is skillful, then illusion and reality become the same.

This is a realm that quickly becomes ethically tricky. There's nothing wrong with taking an herbal supplement to ease your arthritis or your chronic headaches. But somehow there is something wrong with getting rich by lying to people about the pills you are selling. A few years ago, some supplement makers got into hot water because tests revealed that their garlic pills turned out to contain not garlic but rice powder. The pills were having the same placebo effect as before, but somehow consumers felt cheated. I can't resolve this paradox any more than I can explain it. Con men have been with us since the time of Hippocrates, and a part of us has hated them for their ability to trick us—even if it's for our own good.

In the end, it comes down to finding balance. There's nothing wrong with trying your hand at tapping into your brain's medicine cabinet. But if you're not careful, self-healing can be dangerous—even lethal. Here are four handy rules to keep in mind before you start experimenting with the pharmacology of expectation.

Rule #1: Don't endanger yourself. Some alternative health remedies are physically dangerous. Mercury is a poison, chiropractic treatment can seriously damage your spine, and a careless hypnotist can implant terrifying memories that may not be yours.

Also, remember that the supplements industry is not regulated by the FDA or any other government body the way the pharmaceutical industry is. In early 2015, the New York State attorney general investigated a few of the plant supplements for sale at GNC, Target, Walgreens, and Walmart. Forty-five percent of the pills contained no plant matter at all; 33 percent contained something different from what was on the label; and just 22 percent actually tested positive for the plant that was supposed to be in the bottle. Another study out of Canada revealed much the same result, with 60 percent of the supplements containing additives not mentioned on the label, and just

2 of the 12 investigated companies delivering what they claimed. Echinacea, for instance, occasionally contained rice or DNA from pine trees or the buttercup family, but mostly contained no plant DNA at all. Ginkgo biloba similarly contained no ginkgo DNA. Nor did Saint-John's-wort. Nor did ginseng. Chances are you won't ingest poisons, but it's totally possible to take something you might be allergic to without knowing it. Or perhaps, as with some erectile supplements, there will be an active chemical in the mix that's not listed on the packaging that contains unusually high doses.

But there is a far more common way to endanger yourself. If you have a life-threatening disease, do not rely solely on alternative techniques that you suspect might work as placebos. By all means, if you think you might be suggestible, try combining mainstream medicine with alternative therapies to treat the pain, nausea, or depression that might accompany either a disease or its treatment. But as soon as your shaman, homeopath, or acupuncturist suggests you stop using scientifically proven techniques, they are putting you in serious danger.

Choosing between your values and the best path toward health can be difficult. One person who confronted this scenario was Steve Jobs. He spent nine months using a juice-extract therapy to treat his pancreatic cancer before finally seeking conventional treatment. By then it was too late. Of course, it was his second round of cancer, so his prognosis was bad already. And certainly anyone should have the choice to die with dignity. But if your chances are even moderately good with conventional treatment, don't play games with suggestibility.

Rule #2: Don't go broke. It's true that more expensive placebos work better than cheaper ones, but there is a limit. Ranjana Srivastava, an author and oncologist in Melbourne, Australia, has written about the challenges of treating cancer and the relationship between doctor and patient. Her patients have spent thousands on vitamin infusions, smoke therapies, and lavender extracts. She says patients regularly come to her broke and near death after chasing placebos that haven't worked out.

"People [come in] emaciated. They have been robbed physically and financially of their resources," she says. "And the more money you spend on these things, the more defensive you become about it."

One of Srivastava's patients, a retired man on a fixed income and savings, came to her after months of $350 sessions for vitamin infusions. It was his second time fighting prostate cancer, and he just couldn't face the pain and instability of another grueling barrage of chemotherapy. So he spent about $40,000 on promises of miracle cures until the discomfort became so strong that he swallowed his pride and went to a doctor in time to undergo a treatment that worked. Others were not so lucky.

If a cure seems based, in part, on your own suggestibility, then it may be worth it to spend a few bucks every week for some relief. But when you have to stretch your finances to get one special treatment, one weekend meditation with a particular shaman, or a certain top-of-the-line alternative therapy, then you are being played by your own brain.

Rule #3: Don't send any creature to extinction. When I spoke to traditional Chinese medicine practitioner Zhang Lin in Beijing, she said many times that the spirit of an ingredient is more important than its chemistry. She believes materials have an essence beyond what we can see. This may seem like mystic wisdom, and indeed it does have a nice ring to it (it's the kind of thing I would have stuck to the wall of my college dorm room under a picture of the mountains at sunset). But Zhang wasn't talking about the inexorable quality of the human spirit or the intrinsic value of courage; she was referring to a rhinoceros horn. Although a rhino horn might appear to a biochemist as nothing more than a massive fingernail (both substances are composed mostly of a protein called keratin), Zhang tells me it contains the power to break a fever.[31]

Although some species of rhino are assuredly in danger of extinction, rhino horn most assuredly has no medical value. No human condition, however placebo prone, is so serious that another creature deserves to disappear from Earth in the name of maintaining a medical illusion.

Rule #4: Know thyself. As we have seen, for many people the suspicion that a treatment might be a placebo does not change its ability to heal. There's nothing wrong with wondering in the back of your mind whether the herbal immune-boosting shake in front of you is nothing more than a placebo wrapped in wheatgrass puree. But if you want to get the most out of your suggestibility, be strategic about how you approach the damn thing.

First of all, know what kind of person you are. Are you someone who might be suggestible to the power of a certain placebo? If so, what kind? I know I respond to anything fizzy. One of the most powerful placebos for me is Airborne, a cold remedy tablet that dissolves in water with an impressive fizz. Mostly it's just vitamin C, which I could easily get from orange juice. But that wouldn't give me the fizzy magic I crave. Perhaps it reminds me of the OJ-and-7Up drinks I had whenever I was sick as a kid. Perhaps I just like bubbles. But every time I'm fighting off a cold, I reach for Airborne, knowing full well it performs no better than a placebo in double-blind trials. But it always makes me feel better.

---

31 It's widely assumed in the West that in TCM, rhino horns have something to do with penis enhancement or erectile dysfunction, thanks to their phallic shape. But no, Zhang corrected me: The proper use is for fevers.

Second, get to know your condition (or symptoms, if you prefer). Is this a problem that taps into dopamine and expectation? Is it something that modern medicine struggles to treat? By now you should know the list of usual suspects: chronic pain, irritable bowel syndrome, anxiety, nausea, mild depression, headaches, arthritis, fibromyalgia, neuralgia, Parkinson's disease, and addiction. And if you're feeling particularly suggestible, maybe colds, insomnia, weight loss, and athletic performance could also apply. It's possible there are dozens or even hundreds of conditions to add to this list, but for that we'd need to better understand the relationship between belief and the body.

While you are getting to know yourself, try to determine how suggestible you are. If you are looking to cure a physical problem, quit smoking, or beat depression, give hypnosis a try to see if you are hypnotically susceptible. If you are, hold on to that information, like your blood type or your vaccination records. It's a tool that you can use to find relief and improve your life.

Finding a good hypnotist, however, can be tricky. There is no widely accepted certification for hypnosis—a person can call himself a hypnotist after a weekend of trying to learn how. I myself learned to do it while writing this book, but you sure as hell wouldn't pay me to hypnotize you. Mark Jensen, the hypnosis researcher at the University of Washington, says the best thing to do is find someone who is licensed in their profession and uses hypnosis as only one tool. If you are treating pain, go to a specialist who has hypnosis in her repertoire, rather than a pure hypnotist. Many people use hypnosis to make dental work easier—but if you go this route, you should find someone who's a dentist first (perhaps through a professional association's website). This is not to say there aren't plenty of good pure hypnotists out there; it's just that there are also a lot of quacks.

But the minute someone, whether a licensed therapist or your next-door neighbor who dabbles in hypnosis, suggests they can help you retrieve lost memories or improve a memory you do have, walk away. Be careful with techniques like past-life regression or regression to the womb—anything where you'd be retrieving memories you did not have before. Tricking your mind to feel less pain is good sense. Tricking your mind to quit smoking is a great way to prolong your life. But tricking your mind to see something that you're not sure happened is playing with fire.

• • •

As we have seen, suggestibility can have a hell of an effect on a hell of a lot of medical conditions. But not all of them. This is the most fascinating part of the story. Although Parkinson's responds well to placebos, Alzheimer's does not. (Some have even suggested that the very nature of Alzheimer's and the damage it causes in the brain actually harm a trigger for the placebo response.) Anxiety responds to placebos, but obsessive-compulsive disorders traditionally do not. And although the pain and nausea of cancer can be eased with placebos, the tumors themselves do not budge.[32] Of course, spontaneous regression—the sudden retreat of a tumor for no obvious reason—exists both inside and outside the hospital and is more common than you might think. But spontaneous regression is not a product of suggestion (at least not that we know of).

Contemplating the elaborate powers of expectation on the body and its history over thousands of years can be overwhelming. The reach of expectation is vast: 2,000 years of traditional Chinese medicine, the millions who buy into homeopathy and acupuncture, the

---

32 Though it should be said that not nearly enough FDA-approved cancer treatments have gotten the scrutiny they probably deserve. Few are regularly tested in double-blind trials against placebos. Of course, there is an ethical dilemma with giving a placebo to a cancer patient.

trillions of dollars spent by pharmaceutical companies trying to beat the placebo effect. When you step into a televangelist's megachurch and notice he is relying on hypnotic techniques, or when you hear stories of cathartic experiences that sound suspiciously like false memories, you can feel crushed under the weight of the uncertainty between who we are and who we think we are.

And yet suggestibility is also terribly small and intimate. As small as a young boy closing his eyes and listening intently for the voice of God. As simple as a caring healer making eye contact and touching his hand. It's the silence between sleep and pain as you lie in the acupuncturist's office with needles up and down your arm. And it's two young people, desperate and alone for one terrible moment, fighting the panic that their infant is dying.

Over the course of writing this book, a part of me genuinely hoped I would find something so odd, so impressive as to be truly unexplainable. An honest-to-God miracle cure. I never found it. The recoveries I came across were, in the end, completely explainable through science. Are you disappointed? Don't be. After all, what is a miracle but an event that's completely unexplainable? And I ask you: Where's the fun in an event that can't be explained? What is there to learn?

Don't get me wrong; despite my inability to find God on a granite wall 20 years ago, I'm not an atheist. I'm not out to prove that magic and healings and God are all dead. Are miracles real? I have no idea. Science is incapable of proving a negative, so there's no way to say that miracles never happen. But the most exciting kinds of questions don't prove a negative; they delve into all the strange little positives. When the Catholic Church investigates miracle healing, the first thing it does is exclude those things that can be explained by science—in other words, by the normal operations in the body. But from my perspective, those are the most fascinating ones. The healings that don't rise to the level of miracle—the miracle-*like* cures that can be explained, understood, and, who knows, maybe used by all of us—are far more interesting than the unexplainable or supernatural.

That's exactly where expectation and suggestibility come in. These are the miracles of placebos and hypnosis and tricks of the prediction machines in our skulls. These are not the miracles of saints and gurus; these are the miracles available for each and every one of us.

And although I never encountered an unexplainable miracle, I did find a trace of what might drive the other kind. A similar theme that comes up again and again in the world of faith healing. The words "faith," "belief," and even "expectation" suggest a vision toward something that hasn't happened but will. And yet the most successful healings I investigated took the view that the healing had already happened. Mike Pauletich said this when he thought back on his recovery from Parkinson's, and so do many Christian healing ministries and even Christian Science. It's one thing to expect that healing *will* happen, but it seems far more effective to expect that it already has. Placebos might be a promise for the future, but they work only once you've ingested them, convinced that they have done their job.

And more power to them. After years of research, I've come to see suggestibility as Mark Jensen did when he called hypnotizable people "talented." If you can truly find relief in treatments that are no more effective than a placebo, if you can cast out fear and depression with just words, then you are lucky indeed. If you are highly hypnotizable and can treat your illness through trance, pat yourself on the back. For decades, the world has seen you as too easily influenced and pharmaceutical companies have been aggravated by you. But no longer. From here on out, call yourself what you are: talented.

And if you are not that sort of person, if you're the sort who stubbornly resists self-healing, it's impossible to understand those who experience it. I've felt faith healings and I've felt placebo manipulations. But I've also watched hypnotizable people go under and thought to myself, "That didn't happen to me. Maybe they're faking it." Similarly, if you are especially suggestible, it's hard to imagine what it's like not to feel a warm sense of healing from crystals or ancient tonics or the passing of hands over your body. The truly suggestible live in a world all their own.

For most of us, suggestibility is a cocktail of genetics, personal beliefs, experience, and personality. The effectiveness of any given suggestion or expectation depends on how well it's packaged, how it relates to your culture, your experience, and what kind of mood you're in that day. There is a reason scientists haven't yet discovered the perfect placebo responder.

● ● ●

I end this journey where I started it, in the church of my childhood. Back to a faith created by a woman who reportedly could perform astounding miracles and who studied under a student of a student of Franz Mesmer himself. Mary Baker Eddy founded Christian Science in Boston, and to me the practice always seemed perfectly suited to that stately old city. I walk across the sprawling, austere concrete plaza of the Christian Science Mother Church in the heart of town and look across its massive reflecting pool as local children in bathing suits run back and forth in the fountain. For a moment I am reminded how very American this religion is. At once radical yet deeply conservative. Thoughtful and inquisitive yet deeply emotional. Sober and puritanical yet totally nuts to outsiders.

Margit Hammerstrom, a veteran Christian Science healer, smiles and waves from across the plaza, and we walk to the Mary Baker Eddy Library for a quiet spot out of the sun. The library is an impressive, cavernous building with vaulted arches within and stone columns without.

When I asked the Mother Church for a practitioner who could discuss the healing power of faith, hers was the only name they gave me, and I quickly see why. Hammerstrom is confident, with short gray hair and piercing eyes that she assiduously keeps locked with mine. Her manner is somehow both intimidating and deeply soothing. She's thoughtful and relaxed and cuts straight to the chase. I like her even before we sit down.

Hammerstrom has been a Christian Scientist all her life and a healer since 1984. Her conviction in the religion began when she was a child in the 1950s, when she nearly lost her sight in elementary school. All at once, her vision became blurry, and one of her eyes became crossed. An optometrist fitted her with glasses that allowed her to see, but even at the age of seven or eight, she thought of that as a temporary solution and set about healing herself through prayer. She struggled with the issue for four years until finally, one day in a movie theater, she wondered why the film was out of focus. She took off her glasses and saw that she no longer needed them. And she never put them on again.

Hammerstrom explains that unlike almost every other form of alternative treatment, Christian Science permeates every aspect of its adherents' lives. "It's so much more than an alternative means of health care," she says. "Christian Scientists feel that this is a way of life. It doesn't just affect their physical bodies. It affects their relationships and their jobs."

A Christian Scientist is constantly aware that the material world is not what it appears to be and makes efforts to achieve a higher, more spiritual way of living. It's not just a matter of refusing aspirin or drinking beer; it's a whole mind-set. As a kid I was always looking to deflect negative suggestion—for example, cold-and-flu-medication commercials or a character becoming ill on a TV show—that could infiltrate my mind and make me sick. (The official recommendation was to change the channel or look away to protect yourself.) And just when I'd manage to relax, one of my classmates would ask, "Hey, aren't you one of those kids who doesn't go to doctors? What happens if you break your arm?" (Even the most devout Christian Scientist would go to a doctor in a case like that. There are exceptions, it turns out, to every rule.)

Unlike most other forms of alternative healing, Hammerstrom continues, Christian Science doesn't work if it's mixed with other treatments. It requires 100 percent faith and 100 percent dedication. So I ask her the question I have asked traditional Chinese doctors and witch doctors and New Age healers across the world: Since suggestibility and placebos are part of every treatment, what percentage of Christian Science healing is simply the body's response to expectation?

"Do I think expectation plays a role in Christian Science healing? Absolutely," Hammerstrom responds. "Does hope—does 'Gee, I really want this to work'—does that play a role? Absolutely it does."

Presuming that perhaps I'm not being clear, I briefly sketch the neural underpinnings of expectations: the biochemistry of placebos and the effect of belief on the brain. Hammerstrom purses her lips and has to admit that the physical brain itself, with its electrical impulses and chemicals, simply doesn't have a place in the religion, although, she offers, she would be pleased for anyone who gained relief from pain and suffering.

"I know it's a real stretch to apply the concept of science to something that to most people is faith-based," she says. "You say that the test of science is that you have a hypothesis you put to the test, and then you draw conclusions for whether or not your hypothesis is correct. My sense is that God's law isn't a hypothesis; it's a rule. I am not applying this science to test whether it's true. I am applying this science to prove that it *is* true."

This is exactly the same logic that all other alternative medicines, shamans, and faith healers across history have used. It's almost the same way Zhang described traditional Chinese medicine. The thing that separates science from faith is that sometimes science is wrong. It's entirely possible that, either through some unknown brain pathway or by the power of God's law, Hammerstrom healed her vision as a small child. It's also possible that the natural prescription of her eyes was much too strong for her, essentially set up for the size of an adult eyeball rather than a child's. And that because of the strain on her eyes trying to compensate, one eye suddenly became crossed (optometrists call this accommodative or convergence excess esotropia). And that over time, as often happens with children, her eyes grew until the problem corrected itself. If indeed this is the case, then it's likely that the glasses she saw as a temporary measure were actually the treatment that helped her body correct the problem. We don't normally think of a couple of pieces of glass or plastic in front of our face as medicine that makes us better, but occasionally that's exactly what they are.

That same logic could apply to my own childhood miracle. It's true that there was a Legionnaire's outbreak that infected 49 people and killed 15 in 1978. But all the cases traced their infection back to a single Los Angeles hospital. There is an irony buried somewhere in there. Not going to the doctor ensured that I would not receive a diagnosis of Legionnaire's disease. But this same distrust of doctors meant that my parents would have no way of knowing either way.

In science we say that the simplest answer tends to be correct. But in faith, whether in TCM or Christian Science, there can only ever be one answer: the one you believed at the start. Talking to Hammerstrom, I feel a little sad there's no room in my childhood religion for David Patterson or Luana Colloca. I see so much that modern medicine could learn from this practitioner. Her bedside manner, confidence, empathy, and communication skills are markedly better than any conventional clinician I've ever visited. But in the end, there's simply no way to bring together faith and science over the course of an afternoon. So I ask Hammerstrom if there's any chance that a Christian Scientist, like other scientists, could ever refine their beliefs to include neuroscience or modern psychology.

"I want to love God with all my heart—and part of that is not to have any other gods. And I think medicine is a god. I think matter is a god. And I realize that's radical and that you might really be offended by that." She says this so warmly and gently that I don't even realize she's just called everything I believe in a false idol.

I eventually say goodbye and walk around the church grounds contemplating belief, faith, and healing. I walk into the church, sit down in one of the pews, and listen to a tour guide tell the story of how Mary Baker Eddy slipped on a patch of ice and healed herself with just her mind and a copy of the Bible. Above the tour guide, carved into the arching stone walls that rise to form a spacious and stunning nave, is a quote that reads, "If a sense of disease produces suffering and a sense of ease antidotes it, disease is mental. Hence the fact in Christian Science that the human mind alone suffers."

There is no mention of Phineas Quimby or Franz Mesmer or Benjamin Franklin. But as the guide speaks, I can't help thinking of them. And of Henry Beecher, Fabrizio Benedetti, Baron Albert von Schrenck-Notzing, Avicenna, and Morton Jellinek and the questions they and many others spent their lives trying to answer.

Christian Scientists, as well as proponents of traditional Chinese medicine, homeopathy, smoke therapy, Reiki massage, and vitamin E supplements, already think they have the answer. Their adherents have felt the truth—the power—of their healing practices themselves. And for that matter, so have all of us in our own way, whether it's faith in God, supplements, or conventional medicine. We are not credulous weaklings, subject to passing fancies. We are tough-minded, skeptical people. We can't be tricked and we can't be conned. The power of energy fields, superdiluted water, stainless steel needles, and the doctor in the white lab coat is real. We've seen it heal. We've seen it change lives and bring loved ones back from the edge of despair and death.

Plenty of very effective treatments over the course of medical history have proved to be nothing more than suggestion. And plenty more will be proved to be so. Already, studies are starting to suggest that many common forms of arthroscopic joint surgery may be no more successful than a sham surgery. Though if that knee operation made it possible to ski again, who are you to question it?

But why should we have to choose between the two? Doctors have so much to learn from shamans, and shamans have a lot to learn from doctors. If I were to tell your physician that there is a drug with no side effects that could add 10, 20, 30 percent more effectiveness to his treatment, his first move would be to his prescription pad. But tell him that the "drug" is an extra 10 minutes of time, a kindly hand on the shoulder, a clear and cogent explanation of his plan for treatment, and far too many doctors today would look right past you.

What if every prospective doctor in medical school had to pass a placebo test? If they couldn't get their degree until they could give a patient a sugar pill that would cure the ailment in question? Imagine if every doctor had to learn to look at his patients the way Margit Hammerstrom does. Imagine if, just for a moment, doctors were required to see their treatment not as a list of chemicals but as a story to be told.

The human mind is an elaborate, ever changing palace. There are grand libraries of memories and sumptuous ballrooms of emotions. There is the unseen maze of servants' areas where millions of unsung brain functions are performed. And like any good palace, there are more than a few hidden doors and secret passageways. Some of us might spend our time in the ballrooms and the libraries, but can we really say that we know our own brains if we haven't at least cracked one door cleverly disguised as a bookcase? If you can find the courage—and the right key—you might just find a whole new way to visit the palace of your mind. Behind its doors are hidden rooms of pharmacies, waves of undulating electrical currents, and constantly shifting photos telling you who you think you are.

Traveling those secret passageways is a skill. In so many ways, our expectations make us who we are. There's no law that says you have to believe every cockeyed notion that comes your way. But don't judge those who indulge in a little creative expectation tweaking. If suggestibility is a skill, maybe it's possible for us all to hone that skill—to train our brains to expect less pain, more ease of movement. To give control to those who feel they've lost it and relief to those who've become lost to their own suffering. To help us run faster and stand atop a mountain free of pain. And maybe even bring a little more joy and understanding into our lives.

It's just a suggestion. Take it or leave it.

APPENDIX

Rapid Induction Analgesia Procedure

Reprinted with permission from the American Journal of Clinical Hypnosis

Hypnotists use many types of stories—or inductions—to bring their patients into a more suggestible trancelike state. The following is an induction designed to relax a person before going into the dentist chair. The idea is that the hypnotist implants a suggestion that whenever the dentist puts her hand on the patient, he becomes relaxed. If you're curious about hypnosis, try it yourself. Just replace the dentist chair references with whatever idea you hope to suggest.

As you're speaking, play with smooth, easy speaking patterns. Tell a story but don't get caught up in the details. The listener should hear the sound of your voice but also feel comfortable letting his mind wander. And don't worry, the worst that can happen is it doesn't work.

Elicitation of Cooperation

I'd like to talk with you for a moment to see if you'd like to feel more comfortable and relaxed than you might expect. Would you like to feel more comfortable than you do right now?

Initiation of Deep Relaxation

I'm quite sure that it will seem to you that I have really done nothing, that nothing has happened at all. You may feel a bit more relaxed, in a moment, but I doubt that you'll notice any other changes. I'd like you to notice, though, if you're surprised by anything else you might notice.

OK, . . . the really best way to feel more comfortable is to just begin by sitting as comfortably as you can right now, go ahead and adjust yourself to the most comfortable position you like . . . that's fine. Now, I'd like you to notice how much more comfortable you can feel by just taking on very big, satisfying deep breath. Go ahead . . . big deep, satisfying breath . . . that's fine. You may already notice how good that feels, how warm your neck and shoulders can feel.

Now then, I'd like you to take four more very deep, very comfortable breaths, and as you exhale, notice just how comfortable your shoulders can become. And notice how comfortable your eyes can feel when they close. And when they close, just let them stay closed. That's right, just notice that. And notice, too, how, when you exhale, you can feel that relaxation beginning to sink in. Good, that's fine.

Now as you continue breathing, comfortably and deeply and rhythmically, all I'd like you to do is to picture in your mind, just imagine a staircase, any kind you like, with 20 steps and you at the top. Now, you don't need to see all 20 steps at once, you can see any or all of the staircase, any way you like. That's fine. Just notice yourself at the top of the staircase, and the step you're on, and any others you like. However you see it is fine. Now, in a moment, but not yet, I'm going to begin to count out loud from one to 20, and as you may already have guessed, as I count each number I'd like you to take a step down that staircase. See yourself stepping down, feel yourself stepping, one step for each number I count. And all you need to do is notice, just notice, how much more comfortable and relaxed you can feel at each step, as you go down the staircase. One step for each number that I count, the larger the number, the farther down the staircase. The farther down the staircase, the more comfortable you can feel. One step for each number. All right, you can begin to get ready.

Now I'm going to begin. One . . . one step down the staircase. Two . . . two steps down the staircase. That's fine. Three . . . three steps down the staircase. And maybe you already notice how much more relaxed you can feel. I wonder if there are places in your body that feel more relaxed than others. Perhaps your shoulders feel more relaxed than your neck. Perhaps your legs feel more relaxed than your arms. I don't know, and it really doesn't matter. All that matters it that you feel comfortable. That's all.

Four . . . four steps down the staircase, perhaps feeling already places in your body beginning to relax. I wonder if the deep relaxing, restful heaviness in your forehead is already across your face, into your mouth and jaw. Down your neck, deep, restful, heavy. Five ... five steps down the staircase, a quarter of the way down and already beginning, perhaps, to really, really enjoy your relaxation and comfort. Six ... six steps down the staircase. Perhaps beginning to notice that the sounds which were distracting become less so. That all the sounds you can hear become a part of your experience of comfort and relaxation. Anything you can notice becomes a part of your experience of comfort and relaxation.

Seven . . . seven steps down the staircase . . . that's fine. Perhaps noticing the heavy, restful, comfortably relaxing feeling spreading down into your shoulders, into your arms. I wonder if you notice one arm feeling heavier than the other. Perhaps your left arm feels a bit heavier than your right. Perhaps your right arm feels heavier than your left. I don't know, perhaps they both feel equally, comfortably heavy. It really doesn't matter. Just letting yourself become more and more away of the comfortable heaviness. Or is it a feeling of lightness? I really don't know and it really doesn't matter.

Eight . . . eight steps down the staircase . . . perhaps noticing that, even as you relax, your heart seems to beat much faster and harder than you might expect, perhaps noticing the tingling in your fingers. Perhaps wondering about the fluttering of your heavy eyelids. Nine . . . nine steps down the staircase, breathing comfortably, slowly, and deeply, restful. Noticing that heaviness really beginning to sink in as you continue to notice the pleasant, restful, comfortable relaxation just spread through your body. Ten . . . ten steps down the staircase, halfway to the bottom of the staircase, wondering perhaps what might be happening, perhaps wondering if anything at all is happening, and yet, knowing that it really doesn't matter. Feeling so pleasantly restful, just continuing to notice the growing, spreading, comfortable relaxation.

Eleven . . . eleven steps down the staircase. Noticing maybe that as you feel increasingly heavy, more and more comfortable, there's nothing to bother you, nothing to disturb you, as you become deeper and deeper relaxed. Twelve . . . twelve steps down the staircase. I wonder if you notice how easily you can hear the sound of my voice. How easily you can understand the words I say with nothing to bother, nothing to disturb. Thirteen . . . thirteen steps down the staircase. Feeling more and more the real enjoyment of this relaxation and comfort. Fourteen . . . fourteen steps down the staircase, noticing perhaps the sinking, restful pleasantness as your body seems to just sink down, deeper and deeper into the chair, with nothing to bother, nothing to disturb, as though the chair holds you comfortably and warm. Fifteen . . . fifteen steps down the staircase, three-quarters of the way down the staircase. Deeper and deeper relaxed, absolutely nothing at all to do but just enjoy yourself. Sixteen . . . sixteen steps down the staircase, wondering perhaps what to experience at the bottom of the staircase and yet knowing how much more ready you already feel to become deeper and deeper relaxed. More and more comfortable, with nothing to bother, nothing to disturb.

Seventeen . . . seventeen steps down the staircase . . . closer and closer to the bottom, perhaps feeling your heart beating harder and harder. Perhaps feeling the heaviness in your arms and legs become even more clearly comfortable. Knowing that nothing really matters except your enjoyment of your experience of comfortable relaxation, with nothing to bother, nothing to disturb. Eighteen . . . eighteen steps down the staircase. Almost to the bottom, with nothing to bother, nothing to disturb as you continue to go deeper and deeper relaxed. Heavy, comfortable, restful, relaxed. Nothing really to do, no one to please, no one to satisfy. Just to notice how very comfortable and heavy you can feel, as you continue to breathe, slowly and comfortably, restfully. Nineteen . . . nineteen steps down the staircase. Almost to the bottom of the staircase. Nothing to bother, nothing to disturb you as you continue to feel more and more comfortable, more and more relaxed, more and more rested, more and more comfortable, just noticing. And now ...

Twenty . . . you're at the bottom of the staircase. Deeply, deeply relaxed, deeper with every breath you take. As I talk to you for a moment about something you already know a lot about: remembering and forgetting. You know a lot about it, because we all do a lot of it, every moment of every day your remember and then you forget so you can remember something else. You can't remember everything, all at once, so you let some memories move quietly back in your mind. I wonder, for instance, if you remember what you had for lunch yesterday. I would guess that, with not too much effort, you can remember what you had for lunch yesterday. And yet, I wonder if you remember what you had for lunch a month ago today. I would guess the effort is really too great to dig up that memory, though of course it is there. Somewhere, deep in the back of your mind. No need to remember, so you don't. And I wonder if you'll be pleased to notice that things we talk about today, with your eyes closed, are things which you'll remember tomorrow, or the next day, or next week. I wonder if you'll decide to let the memory of these things rest quietly in the back of your mind, or if you'll remember gradually, a bit at the a time. Or perhaps all at once, to be again resting in the back of your mind. Perhaps you'll be surprised to notice that the reception room is the place for memory to surface. Perhaps not. Perhaps you'll notice that it is more comfortable to remember on another day altogether. It really doesn't matter, doesn't matter at all. Whatever you do, however you choose to remember is just fine. Absolutely natural. Doesn't matter at all. Whether you remember tomorrow or the next day, whether you remember all at once or gradually, completely or only partially. Whether you let the memory rest quietly and comfortably in the back of your mind, really doesn't matter at all.

I wonder if you'll be pleased to notice that today, and any day, whenever you feel your head resting back against the headrest, when you feel your head resting back like this, you'll feel reminded of how very comfortable you are feeling right now. Even more comfortable than you feel even now. Comfortable, relaxed, nothing to bother, nothing to disturb. I wonder if you'll be reminded of this comfort too, and relaxation, by just noticing the brightness of the light above. Perhaps this comfort and relaxation will come flooding back, quickly and automatically. I don't know exactly how it will seem, I only know, as perhaps you also know, that your experience will seem surprisingly more pleasant, surprisingly more comfortable, surprisingly more restful than you might expect. With nothing to bother, nothing to disturb. Whatever you are able to notice, everything can be a part of your experience of comfortableness, restfulness, and relaxation. Everything you notice can be a part of being absolutely comfortable.

And I want to remind you that whenever [insert name] touches your right shoulder, like this, you'll experience a feeling of being ready to do something. Whenever I touch your right shoulder, like this, or whenever [insert name] touches your right shoulder, like this, you'll experience a feeling of being ready to do something. Perhaps a feeling of being ready to close your eyes. Perhaps a feeling of being ready to be even more comfortable. Perhaps ready to know even more clearly that there's nothing to bother, nothing to disturb. Perhaps ready to become heavy and tired. I don't know. But whenever I touch your right shoulder, like this, you'll experience a feeling. A feeling of being ready to do something. It really doesn't matter. Nothing really matters but your experience of comfort and relaxation. Absolutely deep comfort and relaxation. With nothing to bother and nothing to disturb. That's fine.

And now as you continue to enjoy your comfortable relaxation, I'd like you to notice how very nice it feels to be this way. To really enjoy your own experience, to really enjoy the feelings your body can give you. And in a moment, but not yet, not until you're ready, but in a moment. I'm going to count from one to 20, and as you know, I'd like you feel yourself going back up the steps. One step for each number. You'll have all the time you need. After all, time is relative. Feel yourself slowly and comfortably going back up the steps, one step for each number I count. More alert as you go back up the steps, one step for each number I count. When I reach three, your eyes will be almost ready to open. When I reach two, they will have opened. And when I reach one, you'll be alter, awake, refreshed. Perhaps as though you'd had a nice nap. Alert, refreshed, comfortable. And even though you'll still be very comfortable and relaxed, you'll be alert and feeling very well. Perhaps surprised, but feeling very well. Perhaps ready to be surprised. No hurry, you'll have all the time you need as you begin to go back up these restful steps.

Twenty . . . nineteen . . . fifteen. A quarter of the way back up, more and more and more alert. No rush, plenty of time. Feel yourself becoming more and more alert. Fourteen . . . thirteen . . . twelve . . .

eleven . . . ten. Halfway back up the stairs. More and more alert. Comfortable but more and more alert. Nine . . . that's right, feel yourself becoming more and more alert. Eight . . . seven . . . six . . . five . . . four . . . three. That's right. Two . . . and one. That's right, wide awake, Alert, relaxed, refreshed. That's fine. How do you feel? Relaxed? Comfortable?

Since the subject has been given posthypnotic suggestions as part of the initial hypnotic experience, it is now possible to elicit an even more satisfactory hypnotic state by utilizing one or more of the post-hypnotic cues suggested. Whenever in the future cues are properly given, the subject rapidly and automatically develops a satisfactory hypnotic state and is adequately analgesic for clinical procedures.

Acknowledgments

S O MANY PEOPLE DESERVE my gratitude for this project. Of course I'd like to thank Hilary Black, Allyson Dickman, and the team at National Geographic Books for having faith in me and bringing this book into being. And my editor Linda Carbone for having endless patience with me during our insane revising marathons. And to Susan Lee Cohen, my agent, for sticking with me all the way through from conception to execution. This stuff is a lot harder than it looks.

I'd like to give a special thanks to the Pulitzer Center on Crisis Reporting, not only for its generous support of this project but for the support for me in the past. Without the center, I honestly have no idea what our media world would become. Never stop the work you do.

There are so many brilliant researchers who gave me their time, their trust, and their amazing knowledge. They have all blown my mind more times than I can count, and I am grateful to every one of them. First among them is Tor Wager, whose 2009 talk on the placebo effect first set me on this path. Then there are Kathryn T. Hall, Sean Mackey, David Patterson, Ted Kaptchuk, and Irving Kirsch—all of whose work has inspired me for years and who treated a goofy journalist with more respect than perhaps he deserved. May they all find the answers they so doggedly chase. And thank you to Luana Colloca for, among other things, electrocuting me. It was stimulating.

It's not easy opening your life to a stranger. It demands a trust and openness that I'm sure I don't have. So my deep, heartfelt gratitude goes to Mike Pauletich and Kristin Grace Erickson for sharing their stories with me. And thank you to the countless other chronic disease patients and false-memory victims who spoke with me.

Thank you to the late Franz Mesmer for following a bizarre and wonderful dream. He was utterly wrong in every way, but you've got to respect a guy for going all in.

I am indebted to Sally Ríos Kuri for her tireless work fact-checking, planning, and all-around supporting me, and to Ileana Mondragon as well. Also to Liz Neely, Ellen Xu, and Wang Qian for their assistance in the field. Thank you Dolly Mascareñas for teaching me the magic of *brujoria* and for being an inspiration.

And thank you, of course, to my family for their support. I'd especially like to thank my father, Sandy Vance, for pushing me to question the world around me and for showing me what it means to be a good man. His unending curiosity for religion and truth has been an inspiration for this book. And to my mother, Dee, for reminding me to always bring the fun.

Thank you to Dominic Bracco for being the kind of journalist anyone would be proud to be and the kind of friend I am proud to have. And to Meghan Dhaliwal for letting me try to hypnotize her—more than once—knowing full well what a bad hypnotist I am. Thanks to the unofficial Mexico City freelancers club—Lesley Tellez, Larry Kaplow, and Ben Herrera—for the support and the kick in the ass I needed to get started. And to Mason Inman for sending me papers on placebos literally for years on end. Who does that?

I am indebted to Laurance Doyle, a man who taught me that a sense of wonder for science and God can be the same thing. The universe isn't as old as it used to be, and the stars are closer than anyone thinks. And thank you to Brenda McCowan for encouraging that wonder through her tutelage in all things dolphin behavior.

A deep thank you to John Wilkes and the U.C. Santa Cruz science writers for scooping up a middling biologist and making him a writer.

And to Rob Irion for keeping their traditions alive. And to the folks at *California Magazine* and the *Chronicle of Higher Education* for showing me what professional journalism looks like. I am indebted to Pam Weintraub, formerly of *Discover* magazine, for helping me craft the magazine article that kicked off this project, and to *Discover* for believing in me way back when. And, of course, to the National Association of Science Writers for giving me my tribe and for honoring my article on placebos with its Journalism Award for Science Reporting.

And, of course, we all need role models. I am deeply indebted to Jamie Shreeve for bringing me into the National Geographic fold and believing in my abilities. I should be lucky to be half the writer he is. I'd like to thank Martha Mendoza, Seth Mnookin, Carl Zimmer, Doug Fox, Annie Finkbeiner, Sara Solovitch, Azam Ahmed, Mike Weissenstein, Alfredo Corchado, Nick Casey, and Dudley Althaus for being the most inspirational journalists I know. If only all media had their integrity and skill.

Finally, I'd like to thank my son, Sebastian Vance. He can't talk yet, but he doesn't need to. His smile is inspiration enough.

Sources

Introduction

Bartram, Jamie. *Legionella and the Prevention of Legionellosis*. World Health Organization, 2007.

Dennett, Daniel C. *Kinds of Minds: Toward an Understanding of Consciousness*. Basic Books, 2008.

First Church of Christ, Scientist. "An Empirical Analysis of Medical Evidence in Christian Science Testimonies of Healing, 1969–1988." Christian Science Board of Directors. (1989): 110–127.

United States Department of Labor. "Legionnaires' Disease." Accessed April 16, 2016. https://www.osha.gov/dts/osta/otm/legionnaires/disease_rec.html.

Chapter 1

Académie Nationale de Médecine. *Report of the Experiments on Animal Magnetism: Made by a Committee of the Medical Section of the French Royal Academy of Sciences—Read at the Meeting of the 21st and 28th of June, 1831*. R. Caddell, 1833.

Ader, R., and N. Cohen. "Behaviorally Conditioned Immunosuppression." *Psychosomatic Medicine* 37, no. 4 (August 1975): 333–40.

Anderson, T. "Dental Treatment in Medieval England." *British Dental Journal* 197, no. 7 (October 9, 2004): 419–25. doi:10.1038/sj.bdj.4811723.

Bañuelos, Nidia. "All Americans Will Pull Together: The Federal Government's Evolving Role in Dealing With Disaster—Thalidomide Drug Crisis 1960s." Robert W. Woodruff Library, Emory University

Libraries. Accessed April 18, 2016. http://guides.main.library.emory. edu/c.php?g=50422&p=325039.

Beecher, Henry. K. "Ethics and Clinical Research. 1966." *Bulletin of the World Health Organization* 79, no. 4 (2001): 367–72.

Beecher, Henry K. "Pain in Men Wounded in Battle." *Annals of Surgery* 123, no. 1 (January 1946): 96–105.

Beecher, Henry K. "The Powerful Placebo." *Journal of the American Medical Association* 159, no. 17 (December 24, 1955): 1602–6.

Brayboy, Coty, and Lakhani, Nirav. "Healing Practices." University of North Carolina "Native American Tribal Studies" exhibit. Accessed April 17, 2016. http://lumbee.web.unc.edu/online-exhibits-2/healing-practices/

Casey, P. A., and R. L. Wynia. *Culturally Significant Plants.* Accessed April 16, 2016. United States Department of Agriculture–Natural Resources Conservation Service, Kansas Plant Materials Center. http://www.nrcs.usda.gov/Internet/FSE_PLANTMATERIALS/ publications/kspmcpu9871.pdf.

de Craen, A. J., P. J. Roos, A. Leonard de Vries, and J. Kleijnen. "Effect of Colour of Drugs: Systematic Review of Perceived Effect of Drugs and of Their Effectiveness." *British Medical Journal* 313, no. 7072 (December 21, 1996): 1624–26.

de Craen, A. J., T. J. Kaptchuk, J. G. Tijssen, and J. Kleijnen. "Placebos and Placebo Effects in Medicine: Historical Overview." *Journal of the Royal Society of Medicine* 92, no. 10 (October 1999): 511–15.

Dixon, Michael, and Kieran Sweeney. *The Human Effect in Medicine: Theory, Research and Practice.* Radcliffe Publishing, 2000.

Ernst, Edzard. "Homeopathy: What Does the 'Best' Evidence Tell Us?" *Medical Journal of Australia* 192, no. 8 (April 19, 2010): 458–60.

Ernst, Edzard. "Is Homeopathy a Clinically Valuable Approach?" *Trends in Pharmacological Sciences* 26, no. 11 (November 2005): 547–48. doi:10.1016/j.tips.2005.09.003.

Gaius, Plinius Secundus. "Pliny the Elder, the Natural History, Book XXVIII. Remedies Derived From Living Creatures. Chap. 18.— Remedies Derived From the Urine." Accessed April 17, 2016. http://www.perseus.tufts.edu/hopper/ text?doc=Perseus%3Atext%3A1999.02.0137%3A- book%3D28%3Achapter%3D18.

James Lind Library. "Louis Lasagna (1923–2003)." Accessed May 6, 2016. http://www.jameslindlibrary.org/articles/louis-lasagna- 1923-2003.

Jellinek, E. M. "Clinical Tests on Comparative Effectiveness of Analgesic Drugs." *Biometrics* 2, no. 5 (October 1946): 87–91.

Jensen, Karin B., Ted J. Kaptchuk, Irving Kirsch, Jacqueline Raicek, Kara M. Lindstrom, Chantal Berna, Randy L. Gollub, Martin Ingvar, and Jian Kong. "Nonconscious Activation of Placebo and Nocebo Pain Responses." *Proceedings of the National Academy of Sciences* 109, no. 39 (September 25, 2012): 15959–64. doi:10.1073/ pnas.1202056109.

Jensen, Karin, Irving Kirsch, Sara Odmalm, Ted J. Kaptchuk, and Martin Ingvar. "Classical Conditioning of Analgesic and Hyperalgesic Pain Responses Without Conscious Awareness." *Proceedings of the National Academy of Sciences of the United States of America* 112, no. 25 (June 23, 2015): 7863–67. doi:10.1073/pnas .1504567112.

Jussieu, Antoine Laurent de. *Rapport de l'un des commissaires chargés par le roi, de l'examen du magnétisme animal.* Herissant, 1784.

Kaptchuk, Ted J., Elizabeth Friedlander, John M. Kelley, M. Norma Sanchez, Efi Kokkotou, Joyce P. Singer, Magda Kowalczykowski, Franklin G. Miller, Irving Kirsch, and Anthony J. Lembo. "Placebos Without Deception: A Randomized Controlled Trial in Irritable Bowel Syndrome." *PLOS ONE* 5, no. 12 (2010): e15591. doi:10.1371/journal.pone.0015591.

Kong, Jian, Rosa Spaeth, Amanda Cook, Irving Kirsch, Brian Claggett, Mark Vangel, Randy L. Gollub, Jordan W. Smoller, and Ted J. Kaptchuk. "Are All Placebo Effects Equal? Placebo Pills, Sham Acupuncture, Cue Conditioning and Their Association." *PLOS ONE* 8, no. 7 (July 31, 2013): e67485. doi:10.1371/journal.pone.0067485.

Loudon, Irvine. "A Brief History of Homeopathy." *Journal of the Royal Society of Medicine* 99, no. 12 (December 2006): 607–10.

McCoy, Alfred W. "Science in Dachau's Shadow: Hebb, Beecher, and the Development of CIA Psychological Torture and Modern Medical Ethics." *Journal of the History of the Behavioral Sciences* 43, no. 4 (2007): 401–17. doi:10.1002/jhbs.20271.

Milne, Iain. "Who Was James Lind, and What Exactly Did He Achieve." *Journal of the Royal Society of Medicine* 105, no. 12 (December 2012): 503–8. doi:10.1258/jrsm.2012.12k090.

Moerman, Daniel E. *Meaning, Medicine and the "Placebo Effect."* Cambridge University Press, 2002.

Murphy, Helen. "A History of Gruesome Medical Cures." *HubPages.* Accessed April 17, 2016. http://hubpages.com/education/A-History-of-Gruesome-Cures.

Nejabat, M., B. Maleki, M. Nimrouzi, A. Mahbodi, and A. Salehi. "Avicenna and Cataracts: A New Analysis of Contributions to Diagnosis and Treatment from the Canon." *Iranian Red Crescent Medical Journal* 14, no. 5 (May 2012): 265–70.

Pacheco-López, Gustavo, Harald Engler, Maj-Britt Niemi, and Manfred Schedlowski. "Expectations and Associations That Heal: Immunomodulatory Placebo Effects and Its Neurobiology." *Brain, Behavior, and Immunity* 20, no. 5 (September 2006): 430–46. doi:10.1016/j.bbi.2006.05.003.

Saljoughian, Payam, and Saljoughian Manouchehr. "The Placebo Effect: Usage, Mechanisms, and Legality." Accessed April 17, 2016. http://www.uspharmacist.com/content/d/in-service/c/31469.

Smith, Cedric M. "Origin and Uses of Primum Non Nocere—Above All, Do No Harm!" *Journal of Clinical Pharmacology* 45, no. 4 (April 2005): 371–77. doi:10.1177/0091270004273680.

United States Food and Drug Administration. "50 Years: The Kefauver-Harris Amendments." Accessed May 6, 2016. http://www.fda.gov/Drugs/NewsEvents/ucm320924.htm.

United States Food and Drug Administration. "Overviews on FDA History: FDA and Clinical Drug Trials—A Short History." Accessed May 6, 2016. http://www.fda.gov/AboutFDA/WhatWeDo/History/Overviews/ucm304485.htm.

Yapijakis, Christos. "Hippocrates of Kos, the Father of Clinical Medicine, and Asclepiades of Bithynia, the Father of Molecular Medicine." *In Vivo* 23, no. 4 (July 1, 2009): 507–14.

Chapter 2

Chapin, Heather, Epifanio Bagarinao, and Sean Mackey. "Real-Time fMRI Applied to Pain Management." *Neuroscience Letters* 520, no. 2 (June 29, 2012): 174–81. doi:10.1016/j.neulet.2012.02.076.

Colloca, Luana, Daniel S. Pine, Monique Ernst, Franklin G. Miller, and Christian Grillon. "Vasopressin Boosts Placebo Analgesic Effects in Women: A Randomized Trial." *Biological Psychiatry*, August 4, 2015. doi:10.1016/j.biopsych.2015.07.019.

Hughes, J., T. W. Smith, H. W. Kosterlitz, Linda A. Fothergill, B. A. Morgan, and H. R. Morris. "Identification of Two Related Pentapeptides From the Brain With Potent Opiate Agonist Activity." *Nature* 258, no. 5536 (December 18, 1975): 577–79. doi:10.1038/258577a0.

Institute of Medicine, Committee on Advancing Pain Research and Education. *Relieving Pain in America: A Blueprint for Transforming Prevention, Care, Education, and Research.* National Academies Press, 2011.

Jensen, Karin, Irving Kirsch, Sara Odmalm, Ted J. Kaptchuk, and Martin Ingvar. "Classical Conditioning of Analgesic and Hyperalgesic Pain Responses Without Conscious Awareness." *Proceedings of the National Academy of Sciences of the United States of America* 112, no. 25 (June 23, 2015): 7863–67. doi:10.1073/pnas.1504567112.

Kaptchuk, Ted J., Elizabeth Friedlander, John M. Kelley, M. Norma Sanchez, Efi Kokkotou, Joyce P. Singer, Magda Kowalczykowski, Franklin G. Miller, Irving Kirsch, and Anthony J. Lembo. "Placebos Without Deception: A Randomized Controlled Trial in Irritable Bowel Syndrome." *PLOS ONE* 5, no. 12 (December 2010): e15591. doi:10.1371/journal.pone.0015591.

Koban, Leonie, and Tor D. Wager. "Beyond Conformity: Social Influences on Pain Reports and Physiology." *Emotion* 16, no. 1 (February 2016): 24–32. doi:10.1037/emo0000087.

Levine, J. D., N. C. Gordon, J. C. Bornstein, and H. L. Fields. "Role of Pain in Placebo Analgesia." *Proceedings of the National Academy of Sciences of the United States of America* 76, no. 7 (July 1979): 3528–31.

Levinovitz, Alan, and Jim Newell. "Chairman Mao Invented Traditional Chinese Medicine." *Slate*, October 22, 2013. http://www.slate.com/articles/health_and_science/medical_examiner/2013/10/traditional_chinese_medicine_origins_mao_invented_it_but_didn_t_believe.2.html.

Lidstone, Sarah C., Michael Schulzer, Katherine Dinelle, Edwin Mak, Vesna Sossi, Thomas J. Ruth, Raul de la Fuente-Fernández, Anthony G. Phillips, and A. Jon Stoessl. "Effects of Expectation on Placebo-Induced Dopamine Release in Parkinson Disease." *Archives of General Psychiatry* 67, no. 8 (August 2010): 857–65. doi:10.1001/archgenpsychiatry.2010.88.

National Institutes of Health. "NIH Clinical Center: 50th Anniversary, 1953–2003." Accessed April 20, 2016. http://clinicalcenter.nih.gov/about/news/anniver50/opening.shtml.

National Institutes of Health. "NIH Clinical Center: Patient Recruitment at the NIH Clinical Center." Accessed April 18, 2016. http://www.cc.nih.gov/recruit/index.html.

Petrovic, Predrag, Eija Kalso, Karl Magnus Petersson, and Martin Ingvar. "Placebo and Opioid Analgesia: Imaging a Shared Neuronal Network." *Science* 295, no. 5560 (March 1, 2002): 1737–40. doi:10.1126/science.1067176.

Ramachandran, V.S., and Eric L. Altschuler. "The Use of Visual Feedback, in Particular Mirror Visual Feedback, in Restoring Brain Function." Accessed April 21, 2016. http://cbc.ucsd.edu/pdf/rama_brain.pdf.

Wager, Tor D., James K. Rilling, Edward E. Smith, Alex Sokolik, Kenneth L. Casey, Richard J. Davidson, Stephen M. Kosslyn, Robert M. Rose, and Jonathan D. Cohen. "Placebo-Induced Changes in fFMRI in the Anticipation and Experience of Pain." *Science* 303, no. 5661 (February 20, 2004): 1162–67. doi:10.1126/science.1093065.

Wilkinson, Missy. "Opium-Soaked Tampons Are the Thing Your Great-Great-Grandparents Hid From You." *Gambit*. Accessed April 20, 2016. http://www.bestofneworleans.com/blogofneworleans/archives/2011/12/02/opium-soaked-tampons-are-the-thing-your-great-great-grandparents-hid-from-you.

Woods, Joycelyn. "Discovery of Endorphines." Accessed April 20, 2016. http://www.methadone.org/library/woods_1994_endorphin.html.

World Health Organization. "Malaria: Q&A on Artemisinin Resistance." Accessed April 21, 2016. http://who.int/malaria/media/artemisinin_resistance_qa/en.

Younger, Jarred, Arthur Aron, Sara Parke, Neil Chatterjee, and Sean Mackey. "Viewing Pictures of a Romantic Partner Reduces Experimental Pain: Involvement of Neural Reward Systems." *PLOS ONE* 5, no. 10 (2010): e13309. doi:10.1371/journal.pone.0013309.

Chapter 3

Bartus, Raymond T., Marc S. Weinberg, and R. Jude Samulski. "Parkinson's Disease Gene Therapy: Success by Design Meets Failure by Efficacy." *Molecular Therapy* 22, no. 3 (March 2014): 487–97. doi:10.1038/mt.2013.281.

Brockner, J., and W. C. Swap. "Resolving the Relationships Between Placebos, Misattribution, and Insomnia: An Individual-Differences Perspective." *Journal of Personality and Social Psychology* 45, no. 1 (July 1983): 32–42.

Bryson, Ethan O., and Elizabeth A. M. Frost. *Perioperative Addiction: Clinical Management of the Addicted Patient.* Springer Science and Business Media, 2011.

Buckenmaier III, Chester. "It's Far More Important to Know What Person the Disease Has Than What Disease the Person Has." *U.S. Medicine.* Accessed April 21, 2016. http://www.usmedicine.com/editor-in-chief/its-far-more-important-to-know-what-person-the-disease-has-than-what-disease-the-person-has.

Ducci, Francesca, and David Goldman. "The Genetic Basis of Addictive Disorders." *Psychiatric Clinics of North America* 35, no. 2 (June 2012): 495–519. doi:10.1016/j.psc.2012.03.010.

Fisher, Seymour, and Rhoda L. Fisher. "Placebo Response and Acquiescence." *Psychopharmacologia* 4, no. 4 (July 1963): 298–301. doi:10.1007/BF00408185.

Gallahan, W. C., D. Case, and R. S. Bloomfeld. "An Analysis of the Placebo Effect in Crohn's Disease Over Time." *Alimentary Pharmacology and Therapeutics* 31, no. 1 (January 2010): 102–7. doi:10.1111/j.1365-2036.2009.04125.x.

Goetz, Christopher. "The Placebo Effect, How It Complicates Parkinson's Disease Research." Parkinson's Disease Foundation." Accessed May 7, 2016. http://www.pdf.org/summer12_placebo.

Goyal M. K., N. Kuppermann, S. D. Cleary, S. J. Teach, and J. M. Chamberlain. "Racial Disparities in Pain Management of Children With Appendicitis in Emergency Departments." *JAMA Pediatrics* 169, no. 11 (November 1, 2015): 996–1002. doi:10.1001/jamapediatrics.2015.1915.

Hall, Kathryn T., Anthony J. Lembo, Irving Kirsch, Dimitrios C. Ziogas, Jeffrey Douaiher, Karin B. Jensen, Lisa A. Conboy, John M. Kelley, Efi Kokkotou, and Ted J. Kaptchuk. "Catechol-O-Methyltransferase val158met Polymorphism Predicts Placebo Effect in Irritable Bowel Syndrome." *PLOS ONE* 7, no. 10 (October 23, 2012): e48135. doi:10.1371/journal.pone.0048135.

Hall, Kathryn T., Christopher P. Nelson, Roger B. Davis, Julie E. Buring, Irving Kirsch, Murray A. Mittleman, Joseph Loscalzo, et al. "Polymorphisms in Catechol-O-Methyltransferase Modify Treatment Effects of Aspirin on Risk of Cardiovascular Disease." *Arteriosclerosis, Thrombosis, and Vascular Biology* 34, no. 9 (September 2014): 2160–67. doi:10.1161/ATVBAHA.114.303845.

Hall, Kathryn T., Joseph Loscalzo, and Ted J. Kaptchuk. "Genetics and the Placebo Effect: The Placebome." *Trends in Molecular Medicine* 21, no. 5 (May 2015): 285–94. doi:10.1016/j.molmed.2015.02.009.

Hosák, Ladislav. "Role of the COMT Gene Val158Met Polymorphism in Mental Disorders: A Review." *European Psychiatry* 22, no. 5 (July 2007): 276–81. doi:10.1016/j.eurpsy.2007.02.002.

Hygen, Beate Wold, Jay Belsky, Frode Stenseng, Stian Lydersen, Ismail Cuneyt Guzey, and Lars Wichstrøm. "Child Exposure to Serious Life Events, COMT, and Aggression: Testing Differential Susceptibility Theory." *Developmental Psychology* 51, no. 8 (2015): 1098–104. doi:10.1037/dev0000020.

Massat, I., D. Souery, J. Del-Favero, M. Nothen, D. Blackwood, W. Muir, R. Kaneva, et al. "Association Between COMT (Val158Met)

Functional Polymorphism and Early Onset in Patients With Major Depressive Disorder in a European Multicenter Genetic Association Study." *Molecular Psychiatry* 10, no. 6 (December 7, 2004): 598–605. doi:10.1038/sj.mp.4001615.

McCambridge, Jim, John Witton, and Diana R. Elbourne. "Systematic Review of the Hawthorne Effect: New Concepts Are Needed to Study Research Participation Effects." *Journal of Clinical Epidemiology* 67, no. 3 (March 2014): 267–77. doi:10.1016/j.jclinepi.2013.08.015.

Nederhof, Anton J. "Methods of Coping With Social Desirability Bias: A Review." *European Journal of Social Psychology* 15, no. 3 (July 1, 1985): 263–80. doi:10.1002/ejsp.2420150303.

Olanow, C. Warren, Raymond T. Bartus, Tiffany L. Baumann, Stewart Factor, Nicholas Boulis, Mark Stacy, Dennis A. Turner, et al. "Gene Delivery of Neurturin to Putamen and Substantia Nigra in Parkinson Disease: A Double-Blind, Randomized, Controlled Trial." *Annals of Neurology* 78, no. 2 (August 2015): 248–57. doi:10.1002/ana.24436.

Owens, Justine E., and Martha Menard. "The Quantification of Placebo Effects Within a General Model of Health Care Outcomes." *Journal of Alternative and Complementary Medicine* 17, no. 9 (September 2011): 817–21. doi:10.1089/acm.2010.0566.

Samuels, A. S., and C. B. Edisen. "A Study of the Psychiatric Effects of Placebo." *Journal of the Louisiana State Medical Society* 113 (March 1961): 114–17.

Sheiner, Eli Oda, Michael Lifshitz, and Amir Raz. "Placebo Response Correlates With Hypnotic Suggestibility." *Psychology of Consciousness: Theory, Research, and Practice* 2, no. 4, (November 30, 2015). doi:10.1037/cns0000074.

Testa, Maria, Mark T. Fillmore, Jeanette Norris, Antonia Abbey, John J. Curtin, Kenneth E. Leonard, Kristin A. Mariano, et al. "Understanding Alcohol Expectancy Effects: Revisiting the Placebo Condition."

Alcoholism, Clinical and Experimental Research 30, no. 2 (February 2006): 339–48. doi:10.1111/j.1530-0277.2006.00039.x.

Tufts Center for the Study of Drug Development. "Tufts CSDD Assessment of Cost to Develop and Win Marketing Approval for a New Drug Now Published." Accessed April 21, 2016. http://csdd.tufts.edu/news/complete_story/tufts_csdd_rd_cost_study_now_published.

Chapter 4

Adler, Shelley R. *Sleep Paralysis: Night-Mares, Nocebos, and the Mind-Body Connection.* Rutgers University Press, 2011.

American Heart Association. "Is Broken Heart Syndrome Real?" Accessed May 10, 2016. http://www.heart.org/HEARTORG/Conditions/More/Cardiomyopathy/Is-Broken-Heart-Syndrome-Real_UCM_448547_Article.jsp#.VzH1pYR97IV.

Benedetti, F., M. Lanotte, L. Lopiano, and L. Colloca. "When Words Are Painful: Unraveling the Mechanisms of the Nocebo Effect." *Neuroscience* 147, no. 2 (June 29, 2007): 260–71. doi:10.1016/j.neuroscience.2007.02.020.

Bicket, Mark C., Anita Gupta, Charlie H. Brown, and Steven P. Cohen. "Epidural Injections for Spinal Pain: A Systematic Review and Meta-Analysis Evaluating the 'Control' Injections in Randomized Controlled Trials." *Anesthesiology* 119, no. 4 (October 2013): 907–31. doi:10.1097/ALN.0b013e31829c2ddd.

Brodwin, Paul. *Medicine and Morality in Haiti: The Contest for Healing Power.* Cambridge University Press, 1996.

Cannon, Walter B. "'Voodoo' Death." *American Anthropologist* 44, no. 2 (April 6, 1942): 169–81. doi:10.1525/aa.1942.44.2.02a00010.

Centers for Disease Control and Prevention. "Clinical Inquiries Regarding Ebola Virus Disease Received by CDC—United States, July 9–November 15, 2014." Accessed May 4, 2016. http://www.cdc.gov/mmwr/preview/mmwrhtml/mm6349a8.htm.

Collier, Roger. "Imagined Illnesses Can Cause Real Problems for Medical Students." *Canadian Medical Association Journal* 178, no. 7 (March 25, 2008): 820. doi:10.1503/cmaj.080316.

Crichton, Fiona, George Dodd, Gian Schmid, Greg Gamble, and Keith J. Petrie. "Can Expectations Produce Symptoms From Infrasound Associated With Wind Turbines?" *Health Psychology* 33, no. 4 (April 2014): 360–64. doi:10.1037/a0031760.

Crichton, Fiona, George Dodd, Gian Schmid, Greg Gamble, Tim Cundy, and Keith J. Petrie. "The Power of Positive and Negative Expectations to Influence Reported Symptoms and Mood During Exposure to Wind Farm Sound." *Health Psychology* 33, no. 12 (December 2014): 1588–92. doi:10.1037/hea0000037.

Davis, E. Wade. "The Ethnobiology of the Haitian Zombi." *Journal of Ethnopharmacology* 9, no. 1 (November 1, 1983): 85–104. doi:10.1016/0378-8741(83)90029-6.

Faasse, Kate, Tim Cundy, and Keith J. Petrie. "Thyroxine: Anatomy of a Health Scare." *BMJ* 339 (December 29, 2009): b5613. doi:10.1136/bmj.b5613.

Haque, Farhana, Subodh Kumar Kundu, Md Saiful Islam, S. M. Murshid Hasan, Asma Khatun, Partha Sarathi Gope, Zahid Hayat Mahmud, et al. "Outbreak of Mass Sociogenic Illness in a School Feeding Program in Northwest Bangladesh, 2010." *PLOS ONE* 8, no. 11 (2013): e80420. doi:10.1371/journal.pone.0080420.

Kiernan, Ben. "The Cambodian Genocide, 1975–1979." Accessed May 4, 2016. http://www.niod.nl/sites/niod.nl/files/Cambodian%20genocide.pdf.

Littlewood, Roland, and Chavannes Douyon. "Clinical Findings in Three Cases of Zombification." *Lancet* 350, no. 9084 (October 1997): 1094–96. doi:10.1016/S0140-6736(97)04449-8.

Macintyre, Pamela, David Rowbotham, and Suellen Walker. *Clinical Pain Management: Acute Pain.* 2nd ed. CRC Press, 2008.

Mackenzie, John. "The Production of the So-Called 'Rose Cold' by Means of an Artificial Rose." *American Journal of Medical Science* 181 (January 1886): 45–56.

Mary Baker Eddy Library. "The Anecdote of the Man with Cholera on Page 154 of *Science and Health*." Accessed April 1, 2013. http://www.marybakereddylibrary.org/research/the-anecdote-of-the-man-with-cholera-on-page-154-of-science-and-health.

McKay, Mike. "Ghost Haunts a Factory Toilet in Bangladesh, Sends Thousands Into Mass Hysteria." Accessed May 4, 2016. http://weekinweird.com/2013/06/23/ghost-haunts-a-factory-toilet-in-bangladesh-sends-thousands-into-mass-hysteria.

Plys, Cate. "Noriega's Curse." *Chicago Reader.* Accessed May 4, 2016. http://www.chicagoreader.com/chicago/noreigas-curse/Content?oid=878875.

Radford, Ben. "Mystery Illness Closes 57 Schools in Bangladesh." *DNews.* Accessed May 4, 2016. http://news.discovery.com/human/psychology/mystery-illness-closes-57-schools-in-bangladesh-160215.htm.

Rubin, Gjames, Miriam Burns, and Simon Wessely. "Possible Psychological Mechanisms for 'Wind Turbine Syndrome.' On the Windmills of Your Mind." *Noise and Health* 16, no. 69 (2014): 116. doi:10.4103/1463-1741.132099.

Swancer, Brent. "The Mysterious Real Zombies of Haiti." *Mysterious Universe.* Accessed May 4, 2016. http://mysteriousuniverse.org/2014/08/the-mysterious-real-zombies-of-haiti.

Thompson, Dennis. "Americans Increasingly Anxious About Ebola: Poll." *Consumer HealthDay.* Accessed May 4, 2016. https://consumer.healthday.com/mental-health-information-25/emotional-disorder-news-228/americans-increasingly-anxious-about-ebola-poll-692545.html.

Varelmann, Dirk, Carlo Pancaro, Eric C. Cappiello, and William R. Camann. "Nocebo-Induced Hyperalgesia During Local Anesthetic

Injection." *Anesthesia and Analgesia* 110, no. 3 (March 1, 2010): 868–70. doi:10.1213/ANE.0b013e3181cc5727.

Wick, Joshua L. "Warrior Clinic Reduces Pain Medication Use." United States Military. Accessed May 4, 2016. http://www.army .mil/article/55754.

Chapter 5

Bodie W. *The Bodie Book: Hypnotism, Electricity, Mental Suggestion, Magnetic Touch, Clairvoyance, Telepathy.* Wood Library Museum. Accessed May 10, 2016. http://www.woodlibrarymuseum.org/ rarebooks/item/451/bodie-w.-the-bodie-book:-hypnotism,-electric ity,-mental-suggestion,-magnetic-touch,-clairvoyance,-telepathy, -1905.

Braid, James, and Michael Heap. *The Discovery of Hypnosis: The Complete Writings of James Braid, the Father of Hypnotherapy.* Edited by Donald Robertson. National Council for Hypnotherapy, 2009.

Eddy, Mary Baker. *Science and Health, Chapter V: Animal Magnetism Unmasked.* Accessed May 10, 2016. http://christianscience.com/ the-christian-science-pastor/science-and-health/chapter-v-animal- magnetism-unmasked.

Hilgard, Ernest R., André M. Weitzenhoffer, and Philip Gough. "Individual Differences in Susceptibility to Hypnosis." *Proceedings of the National Academy of Sciences of the United States of America* 44, no. 12 (December 15, 1958): 1255–59.

Human Interface Technology Laboratory Projects. "Virtual Reality Pain Reduction." University of Washington and U.W. Harborview Burn Center. Accessed April 27, 2016. https://www.hitl.washing ton.edu/projects/vrpain.

Hypnotism Act, 1952. Accessed April 26, 2016. http://www.legisla tion.gov.uk/ukpga/Geo6and1Eliz2/15-16/46.

Jensen, Mark P., Leslie H. Sherlin, Felipe Fregni, Ann Gianas, Jon D. Howe, and Shahin Hakimian. "Baseline Brain Activity Predicts Response to Neuromodulatory Pain Treatment." *Pain Medicine* 15, no. 12 (December 2014): 2055–63. doi:10.1111/pme.12546.

Jensen, Mark P., Shahin Hakimian, Leslie H. Sherlin, and Felipe Fregni. "New Insights Into Neuromodulatory Approaches for the Treatment of Pain." *Journal of Pain* 9, no. 3 (March 2008): 193–99. doi:10.1016/j.jpain.2007.11.003.

Lafferton, Emese. "Death by Hypnosis: An 1894 Hungarian Case and Its European Reverberations." *Endeavour* 30, no. 2 (June 2006): 65–70. doi:10.1016/j.endeavour.2006.04.005.

Mason, A. A. "Case of Congenital Ichthyosiform Erythrodermia of Brocq Treated by Hypnosis." *British Medical Journal* 2, no. 4781 (August 23, 1952): 422–23.

Mason, A. A. "Ichthyosis and Hypnosis." *British Medical Journal* 2, no. 4930 (July 2, 1955): 57–58.

Prentiss, D. W. "Hypnotism in Animals." *American Naturalist* 16, no. 9 (1882): 715–27.

Rainville, P., G. H. Duncan, D. D. Price, B. Carrier, and M. C. Bushnell. "Pain Affect Encoded in Human Anterior Cingulate but Not Somatosensory Cortex." *Science* 277, no. 5328 (August 15, 1997): 968–71.

Schrenck-Notzing, Albert von. "Phenomena of Materialisation: A Contribution to the Investigation of Mediumistic Teleplastics (1923)." *Public Domain Review.* Accessed April 25, 2016. http://publicdomainreview.org/collections/phenomena-of-materialisation-1923.

Scott, Sir Walter. *Delphi Complete Works of Sir Walter Scott (Illustrated).* Delphi Classics, 2013.

Shor, Ronald E., and Carota. O. E. "Harvard Group Scale of Hypnotic Susceptibility, Form A." Consulting Psychologists Press, 1962.

Sommer, Andreas. "Policing Epistemic Deviance: Albert von Schrenck-Notzing and Albert Moll." *Medical History* 56, no. 2 (April 2012): 255–76. doi:10.1017/mdh.2011.36.

Spiegel, H. "An Eye-Roll Test for Hypnotizability." *American Journal of Clinical Hypnosis* 15, no. 1 (July 1972): 25–28. doi:10.1080/00 029157.1972.10402206.

Tellegen, Auke, and Gilbert Atkinson. "Openness to Absorbing and Self-Altering Experiences ('Absorption'), a Trait Related to Hypnotic Susceptibility." *Journal of Abnormal Psychology* 83, no. 3 (1974): 268–77. doi:10.1037/h0036681.

U.K. College of Hypnosis and Hypnotherapy. "The History of Hypnotism for Childbirth: Excerpt From a Book Chapter by Plantonov." October 22, 2010. http://www.ukhypnosis.com/2010/10/22/ the-history-of-hypnotism-in-childbirth-platonov.

Weitzenhoffer, A. M. and Hilgard, E. R. "Stanford Hypnotic Susceptibility Scale, Form C." Consulting Psychologists Press, 1962.

White, M.M. "The Physical and Mental Traits of Individuals Susceptible to Hypnosis." *Journal of Abnormal and Social Psychology* 25, no. 3 (1930): 293–98. doi:10.1037/h0075216.

Chapter 6

Bernstein, Daniel M., and Elizabeth F. Loftus. "How to Tell If a Particular Memory Is True or False." *Perspectives on Psychological Science* 4, no. 4 (July 1, 2009): 370–74. doi:10.1111/j.1745-6924.2009 .01140.x.

Braun, Kathryn A., Rhiannon Ellis, and Elizabeth F. Loftus. "Make My Memory: How Advertising Can Change Our Memories of the Past." *Psychology and Marketing* 19, no. 1 (January 1, 2002): 1–23. doi:10.1002/mar.1000.

Clancy, Susan A., Richard J. McNally, Daniel L. Schacter, Mark F. Lenzenweger, and Roger K. Pitman. "Memory Distortion in People

Reporting Abduction by Aliens." *Journal of Abnormal Psychology* 111, no. 3 (August 2002): 455–61.

Courtney Hritz, Amelia, Caisa Elizabeth Royer, Rebecca K. Helm, Kayla A. Burd, Karen Ojeda, and Stephen J. Ceci. "Children's Suggestibility Research: Things to Know Before Interviewing a Child." *Anuario de Psicología Jurídica* 25 (2015). http://www.reda-lyc.org/resumen.oa?id=315040291002.

Courts, Committee on Scientific Approaches to Understanding and Maximizing the Validity and Reliability of Eyewitness Identification in Law Enforcement, and Committee on Science and Law, Policy and Global Affairs, Committee on Law and Justice, Division of Behavioral and Social Sciences and Education, and National Research Council. *Identifying the Culprit: Assessing Eyewitness Identification.* National Academies Press, 2015.

Dasse, Michelle N., Gary R. Elkins, and Charles A. Weaver. "Hypnotizability, Not Suggestion, Influences False Memory Development." *International Journal of Clinical and Experimental Hypnosis* 63, no. 1 (2015): 110–28. doi:10.1080/00207144.2014.961880.

Dewhurst, Stephen A., Rachel J. Anderson, and Lauren M. Knott. "A Gender Difference in the False Recall of Negative Words: Women DRM More Than Men." *Cognition and Emotion* 26, no. 1 (2012): 65–74. doi:10.1080/02699931.2011.553037.

Goldstein, Eleanor, and Mark Pendergrast. "The Wrongful Conviction of Bruce Perkins." Accessed April 27, 2016. http://ncrj.org/wp-con tent/uploads/sponsored/Perkins.

Howe, Mark L. "Children (but Not Adults) Can Inhibit False Memories." *Psychological Science* 16, no. 12 (December 1, 2005): 927–31. doi:10.1111/j.1467-9280.2005.01638.x.

Hunt, Kathryn L., and Lars Chittka. "Merging of Long-Term Memories in an Insect." *Current Biology* 25, no. 6 (March 16, 2015): 741–45. doi:10.1016/j.cub.2015.01.023.

Laney, Cara, and Elizabeth F. Loftus. "Recent Advances in False Memory Research." *South African Journal of Psychology* 43, no. 2 (June 1, 2013): 137–46. doi:10.1177/0081246313484236.

Lanning, Kenneth V. *Investigator's Guide to Allegations of "Ritual" Child Abuse.* Behavioral Science Unit, National Center for the Analysis of Violent Crime, Federal Bureau of Investigation, FBI Academy, 1992.

Loftus, E. F., and J. E. Pickrell. "The Formation of False Memories." *Psychiatric Annals 25:12* (December 1995): 720–25.

Loftus, E. F., D. G. Miller, and H. J. Burns. "Semantic Integration of Verbal Information Into a Visual Memory." *Journal of Experimental Psychology: Human Learning and Memory* 4, no. 1 (January 1978): 19–31.

McFarlane, Felicity, Martine B. Powell, and Paul Dudgeon. "An Examination of the Degree to Which IQ, Memory Performance, Socio-Economic Status and Gender Predict Young Children's Suggestibility." *Legal and Criminological Psychology* 7, no. 2 (September 1, 2002): 227–39. doi:10.1348/135532502760274729.

Meyersburg, Cynthia A., Ryan Bogdan, David A. Gallo, and Richard J. McNally. "False Memory Propensity in People Reporting Recovered Memories of Past Lives." *Journal of Abnormal Psychology* 118, no. 2 (May 2009): 399–404. doi:10.1037/a0015371.

Morgan III, C. A., Steven Southwick, George Steffian, Gary A. Hazlett, and Elizabeth F. Loftus. "Misinformation Can Influence Memory for Recently Experienced, Highly Stressful Events." *International Journal of Law and Psychiatry* 36, no. 1 (January 2013): 11–17. doi:10.1016/j.ijlp.2012.11.002.

National Institutes of Health. "PTSD: A Growing Epidemic." *NIH MedlinePlus* 4, no. 1 (Winter 2009): 10–14. Accessed April 27, 2016. https://www.nlm.nih.gov/medlineplus/magazine/issues/winter09/articles/winter09pg10-14.html.

Neisser, Ulric, and Nicole Harsch. "Phantom Flashbulbs: False Recollections of Hearing the News About Challenger." In *Affect and Accuracy in Recall: Studies of "Flashbulb" Memories*, edited by E. Winograd and U. Neisser, 9–31. Emory Symposia in Cognition, 4. Cambridge University Press, 1992.

Okuda, Jiro, Toshikatsu Fujii, Hiroya Ohtake, Takashi Tsukiura, Kazuyo Tanji, Kyoko Suzuki, Ryuta Kawashima, Hiroshi Fukuda, Masatoshi Itoh, and Atsushi Yamadori. "Thinking of the Future and Past: The Roles of the Frontal Pole and the Medial Temporal Lobes." *NeuroImage* 19, no. 4 (August 2003): 1369–80.

Pace-Schott, Edward F., Anne Germain, and Mohammed R. Milad. "Sleep and REM Sleep Disturbance in the Pathophysiology of PTSD: The Role of Extinction Memory." *Biology of Mood and Anxiety Disorders* 5 (2015): 3. doi:10.1186/s13587-015-0018-9.

Patihis, Lawrence, Steven J. Frenda, Aurora K. R. LePort, Nicole Petersen, Rebecca M. Nichols, Craig E. L. Stark, James L. McGaugh, and Elizabeth F. Loftus. "False Memories in Highly Superior Autobiographical Memory Individuals." *Proceedings of the National Academy of Sciences* 110, no. 52 (December 24, 2013): 20947–52. doi:10.1073/pnas.1314373110.

Price, Heather L., and Thomas L. Phenix. "True (but Not False) Memories Are Subject to Retrieval-Induced Forgetting in Children." *Journal of Experimental Child Psychology* 133 (May 2015): 1–15. doi:10.1016/j.jecp.2015.01.009.

Ramirez, Steve, Xu Liu, Pei-Ann Lin, Junghyup Suh, Michele Pignatelli, Roger L. Redondo, Tomás J. Ryan, and Susumu Tonegawa. "Creating a False Memory in the Hippocampus." *Science* 341, no. 6144 (July 26, 2013): 387–91. doi:10.1126/science.1239073.

Reyna, V. F., and C. J. Brainerd. "Fuzzy-Trace Theory and False Memory: New Frontiers." *Journal of Experimental Child Psychology* 71, no. 2 (November 1998): 194–209. doi:10.1006/jecp.1998.2472.

Riba, J., M. Valle, F. Sampedro, A. Rodríguez-Pujadas, S. Martínez-Horta, J. Kulisevsky, and A. Rodríguez-Fornells. "Telling True From False: Cannabis Users Show Increased Susceptibility to False Memories." *Molecular Psychiatry* 20, no. 6 (June 2015): 772–77. doi:10.1038/mp.2015.36.

Roediger, Henry L., Jason M. Watson, Kathleen B. McDermott, and David A. Gallo. "Factors That Determine False Recall: A Multiple Regression Analysis." *Psychonomic Bulletin and Review* 8, no. 3 (September 2001): 385–407. doi:10.3758/BF03196177.

Schacter, Daniel L. *The Seven Sins of Memory: How the Mind Forgets and Remembers.* 1st ed. Mariner Books, 2002.

Zhu, Bi, Chuansheng Chen, Elizabeth F. Loftus, Chongde Lin, Qinghua He, Chunhui Chen, He Li, Gui Xue, Zhonglin Lu, and Qi Dong. "Individual Differences in False Memory From Misinformation: Cognitive Factors." *Memory* 18, no. 5 (July 2010): 543–55. doi:10.1080/09658211.2010.487051.

Chapter 7

Amanzio, M., and F. Benedetti. "Neuropharmacological Dissection of Placebo Analgesia: Expectation-Activated Opioid Systems Versus Conditioning-Activated Specific Subsystems." *Journal of Neuroscience* 19, no. 1 (January 1, 1999): 484–94.

American Society of Addiction Medicine. "Opioid Addiction: 2016 Facts and Figures." Accessed May 2, 2016. http://www.asam.org/docs/default-source/advocacy/opioid-addiction-disease-facts-figures.pdf.

Ariel, Gideon, and William Saville. "Anabolic Steroids: The Physiological Effects of Placebos." *Medicine and Science in Sports and Exercise* 4, no. 2 (1972): 124–26.

Beedie, Christopher J., and Abigail J. Foad. "The Placebo Effect in Sports Performance: A Brief Review." *Sports Medicine* 39, no. 4 (2009): 313–29.

Bradford, Andrea, and Cindy Meston. "Correlates of Placebo Response in the Treatment of Sexual Dysfunction in Women: A Preliminary Report." *Journal of Sexual Medicine* 4, no. 5 (September 2007): 1345–51. doi:10.1111/j.1743-6109.2007.00578.x.

Buscemi, N., B. Vandermeer, C. Friesen, L. Bialy, M. Tubman, M. Ospina, T. P. Klassen, and M. Witmans. "Manifestations and Management of Chronic Insomnia in Adults: Summary." June 2005. http://www.ncbi.nlm.nih.gov/books/NBK11906.

Childress, Anna Rose, Ronald N. Ehrman, Ze Wang, Yin Li, Nathan Sciortino, Jonathan Hakun, William Jens, et al. "Prelude to Passion: Limbic Activation by 'Unseen' Drug and Sexual Cues." *PLOS ONE* 3, no. 1 (2008): e1506. doi:10.1371/journal.pone.0001506.

Cole-Harding, Shirley, and Vicki J. Michels. "Does Expectancy Affect Alcohol Absorption?" *Addictive Behaviors* 32, no. 1 (January 2007): 194–98. doi:10.1016/j.addbeh.2006.03.042.

Colloca, Luana, and Franklin G. Miller. "The Nocebo Effect and Its Relevance for Clinical Practice." *Psychosomatic Medicine* 73, no. 7 (September 2011): 598–603. doi:10.1097/PSY.0b013e31822 94a50.

Corder, G., S. Doolen, R. R. Donahue, M. K. Winter, B. L. Jutras, Y. He, X. Hu, et al. "Constitutive μ-Opioid Receptor Activity Leads to Long-Term Endogenous Analgesia and Dependence." *Science (New York, N.Y.)* 341, no. 6152 (September 20, 2013): 1394–99. doi:10.1126/science.1239403.

Crum, Alia J., and Ellen J. Langer. "Mind-Set Matters: Exercise and the Placebo Effect." *Psychological Science* 18, no. 2 (February 2007): 165–71. doi:10.1111/j.1467-9280.2007.01867.x.

Crum, Alia J., William R. Corbin, Kelly D. Brownell, and Peter Salovey. "Mind Over Milkshakes: Mindsets, Not Just Nutrients, Determine Ghrelin Response." *Health Psychology* 30, no. 4 (July 2011): 424–31. doi:10.1037/a0023467.

Derry, Fadel, Claes Hultling, Allen D. Seftel, and Marca L. Sipski. "Efficacy and Safety of Sildenafil Citrate (Viagra) in Men with Erectile Dysfunction and Spinal Cord Injury: A Review." *Urology* 60, no. 2, Suppl 2 (September 2002): 49–57.

Federal Trade Commission. "Green Coffee Bean Manufacturer Settles FTC Charges of Pushing Its Product Based on Results of 'Seriously Flawed' Weight-Loss Study." Accessed May 2, 2016. https://www.ftc.gov/news-events/press-releases/2014/09/green-coffee-bean-manufacturer-settles-ftc-charges-pushing-its.

Festa, Jessica. "Unusual Aphrodisiacs From Asian Countries." *Gadling*, March 3, 2012. http://gadling.com/2012/03/03/unusual-aphrodisiacs-from-asian-countries.

Haugtvedt, Curtis P., Richard E. Petty, and John T. Cacioppo. "Need for Cognition and Advertising: Understanding the Role of Personality Variables in Consumer Behavior." *Journal of Consumer Psychology* 1, no. 3 (January 1, 1992): 239–60. doi:10.1016/S1057-7408(08)80038-1.

Karlsson, Henry K., Lauri Tuominen, Jetro J. Tuulari, Jussi Hirvonen, Riitta Parkkola, Semi Helin, Paulina Salminen, Pirjo Nuutila, and Lauri Nummenmaa. "Obesity Is Associated With Decreased µ-Opioid but Unaltered Dopamine D2 Receptor Availability in the Brain." *Journal of Neuroscience* 35, no. 9 (March 4, 2015): 3959–65. doi:10.1523/JNEUROSCI.4744-14.2015.

Kasnoff. Craig. "Chinese Medicine." Accessed May 3, 2016. http://www.tigersincrisis.com/traditional_medicine.htm.

Korownyk, Christina, Michael R. Kolber, James McCormack, Vanessa Lam, Kate Overbo, Candra Cotton, Caitlin Finley, et al. "Televised Medical Talk Shows: What They Recommend and the Evidence to Support Their Recommendations: A Prospective Observational Study." *BMJ* 349 (December 17, 2014): g7346. doi:10.1136/bmj.g7346.

Lehmiller, Justin. "Sex Question Friday: Why Can't I Maintain Sexual Interest in One Person?" Sex and Psychology blog. Accessed May 3, 2016. http://www.lehmiller.com/blog/2014/12/19/sex-question-friday-why-cant-i-maintain-sexual-interest-in-one-person.

Lynch, C. D., R. Sundaram, J. M. Maisog, A. M. Sweeney, and G. M. Buck Louis. "Preconception Stress Increases the Risk of Infertility: Results From a Couple-Based Prospective Cohort Study—the LIFE Study." *Human Reproduction* 29, no. 5 (May 2014): 1067–75. doi:10.1093/humrep/deu032.

Mayberg, Helen S., J. Arturo Silva, Steven K. Brannan, Janet L. Tekell, Roderick K. Mahurin, Scott McGinnis, and Paul A. Jerabek. "The Functional Neuroanatomy of the Placebo Effect." *American Journal of Psychiatry* 159, no. 5 (May 1, 2002): 728–37. doi:10.1176/appi.ajp.159.5.728.

National Center for Biotechnology Information. "Sildenafil Citrate." Accessed May 3, 2016. http://www.ncbi.nlm.nih.gov/mesh/?term=UK-92,480-10.

NPR. "'Two-Buck Chuck' Snags Top Wine Prize." Accessed May 2, 2016. http://www.npr.org/templates/story/story.php?storyId=1963794.

Park, Ji Kyung, and Deborah Roedder John. "Got to Get You Into My Life: Do Brand Personalities Rub Off on Consumers?" *Association for Consumer Research* 38. Accessed May 11, 2016. http://www.acrwebsite.org/volumes/15957/volumes/v38/NA-38.

Park, Ji Kyung, and Deborah Roedder John. "I Think I Can, I Think I Can: Brand Use, Self-Efficacy, and Performance." *Journal of Marketing Research* 51, no. 2 (March 5, 2014): 233–47. doi:10.1509/jmr.11.0532.

Perlis, Michael, Michael Grandner, Jarcy Zee, Erin Bremer, Julia Whinnery, Holly Barilla, Priscilla Andalia, et al. "Durability of Treatment Response to Zolpidem With Three Different

Maintenance Regimens: A Preliminary Study." *Sleep Medicine* 16, no. 9 (September 2015): 1160–68. doi:10.1016/j.sleep.2015.06.015.

Ross, Ramzy, Cindy M. Gray, and Jason M. R. Gill. "Effects of an Injected Placebo on Endurance Running Performance." *Medicine and Science in Sports and Exercise* 47, no. 8 (August 2015): 1672–81. doi:10.1249/MSS.0000000000000584.

Substance Abuse and Mental Health Services Administration. "National Survey on Drug Use and Health." Accessed May 11, 2016. https://nsduhweb.rti.org/respweb/homepage.cfm.

Vinson, Joe A, Bryan R Burnham, and Mysore V. Nagendran. "Randomized, Double-Blind, Placebo-Controlled, Linear Dose, Crossover Study to Evaluate the Efficacy and Safety of a Green Coffee Bean Extract in Overweight Subjects." *Diabetes, Metabolic Syndrome and Obesity: Targets and Therapy* 5 (January 18, 2012): 21–27. doi:10.2147/DMSO.S27665.

Chapter 8

Benedetti, Fabrizio, Elisa Carlino, and Antonella Pollo. "How Placebos Change the Patient's Brain." *Neuropsychopharmacology* 36, no. 1 (January 2011): 339–54. doi:10.1038/npp.2010.81.

Chvetzoff, Gisèle, and Ian F. Tannock. "Placebo Effects in Oncology." *Journal of the National Cancer Institute* 95, no. 1 (January 1, 2003): 19–29. doi:10.1093/jnci/95.1.19.

Huppert, Jonathan D., Luke T. Schultz, Edna B. Foa, David H. Barlow, Jonathan R. T. Davidson, Jack M. Gorman, M. Katherine Shear, H. Blair Simpson, and Scott W. Woods. "Differential Response to Placebo Among Patients With Social Phobia, Panic Disorder, and Obsessive-Compulsive Disorder." *American Journal of Psychiatry* 161, no. 8 (August 1, 2004): 1485–87. doi:10.1176/appi.ajp.161.8.1485.

Lewis, C. S., and Kathleen Norris. *Mere Christianity.* Rev. ed. HarperOne, 2015.

New York State Office of the Attorney General. "A.G. Schneiderman Asks Major Retailers to Halt Sales of Certain Herbal Supplements as DNA Tests Fail to Detect Plant Materials Listed on Majority of Products Tested." Accessed May 9, 2016. http://www.ag.ny.gov/press-release/ag-schneiderman-asks-major-retailers-halt-sales-certain-herbal-supplements-dna-tests.

Newmaster, Steven G., Meghan Grguric, Dhivya Shanmughanandhan, Sathishkumar Ramalingam, and Subramanyam Ragupathy. "DNA Barcoding Detects Contamination and Substitution in North American Herbal Products." *BMC Medicine* 11 (2013): 222. doi:10.1186/1741-7015-11-222.

Olshansky, Brian. "Placebo and Nocebo in Cardiovascular Health: Implications for Healthcare, Research, and the Doctor-Patient Relationship." *Journal of the American College of Cardiology* 49, no. 4 (January 30, 2007): 415–21. doi:10.1016/j.jacc.2006.09.036.

Quora. "Why Did Steve Jobs Choose Not to Effectively Treat His Cancer? Accessed May 9, 2016. https://www.quora.com/Why-did-Steve-Jobs-choose-not-to-effectively-treat-his-cancer.